Pregnancy and Birth

THE BEST EVIDENCE

Dr. Joyce Barrett and Teresa Pitman

KEY PORTER BOOKS

For our families: John, Pam and Liza Hambley
Matthew, Lisa, Daniel and Jeremy Pitman

Canadian Cataloguing in Publication Data

Barrett, Joyce, 1944–
      Pregnancy and birth : the best evidence

(A Today's Parent book)
Includes index.
ISBN 1-55263-026-9

1. Pregnancy – Popular works. 2. Prenatal care. 3. Childbirth.
I. Pitman, Teresa. II. Title. III. Series.

RG525.B37 1999   618.2'4   C98-933005-2

The publisher gratefully acknowledges the support of the Canada Council for the Arts and the Ontario Arts Council for its publishing program.

THE CANADA COUNCIL | LE CONSEIL DES ARTS
FOR THE ARTS | DU CANADA
SINCE 1957 | DEPUIS 1957

Key Porter Books Limited
70 The Esplanade
Toronto, Ontario
Canada M5E 1R2

www.keyporter.com

Electronic formatting: Jean Lightfoot Peters
Design: Peter Maher

All illustrations by Karen Visser and reproduced with her permission.

Printed and bound in Canada

99 00 01 02   6 5 4 3 2

Contents

Acknowledgments

We would like to express our appreciation to all those who read sections of the manuscript and gave us their comments, criticisms and suggestions. In particular, we would like to thank Dr. Murray Enkin for his thoughtful feedback and recommendations, and Holly Bennett for her gentle yet persistent editorial guidance. Finally, our thanks to the women who shared their experiences during pregnancy and birth through their letters and in interviews.

Introduction

Why You Should Read This Book

Trish has been waiting all morning to share her news. As the other women from her aerobics class gather for their traditional early-morning snack and chat, she grabs the opportunity to make her announcement.

"Guess what—I'm pregnant!"

"Congratulations!" There is a chorus of excited comments.

Then Rita says, "Have you found an obstetrician yet? Mine was excellent, if you want his name."

Shelley jumps in: "Don't go to an obstetrician! Get a midwife—I had one and she was wonderful—they give you so much support."

Rita shakes her head: "No, you need an obstetrician just in case something goes wrong. They're the experts."

Alana adds, "Well, I wouldn't go with a midwife. I stayed with my family doctor and he was pretty good. I had a huge episiotomy, though, and it still bothers me."

"Sure," says Gwen, "but think about what would have happened if you hadn't had the episiotomy. You'd probably have had a bad tear instead, and everyone knows that's worse."

Shelley disagrees: "My midwife said that isn't true. Most women don't need episiotomies, and she's good at delivering babies without tearing."

Jane turns to Trish and asks, "Are you having an amnio? When's your first ultrasound scheduled?"

Trish shrugs her shoulders. She doesn't even know what an amnio is, and thought ultrasound was something used to detect fish swimming under a boat.

Shelley says, "I didn't have any ultrasounds."

Gwen says, "I had seven. But, of course, I had gestational diabetes so I was high risk."

Rita says, "And make sure you get the epidural as early as possible."

Trish heads off to work with her head full of new questions and concerns. She hadn't known that being pregnant meant making so many decisions.

As a pregnant woman, your conversations

Our Sources

Effective Care in Pregnancy and Childbirth
edited by Iain Chalmers, Murray Enkin and
Marc J.N.C. Keirse
(two volumes) published by Oxford
University Press, 1989

*A Guide to Effective Care in Pregnancy
and Childbirth*
by Murray Enkin, Marc J.N.C. Keirse, Mary
Renfrew and James Neilson
published by Oxford University Press, 1995

The Cochrane Library
published by Update Software, disk format,
updated frequently

with other mothers are guaranteed to reveal different opinions about almost every aspect of pregnancy and childbirth. Every woman you talk to will have a different birth story—and that's understandable, because every pregnancy and every birth is unique. (Yours will be, too!) But you may find yourself feeling very confused by the dramatically different ideas you're hearing about everything from prenatal tests to how to take care of a newborn.

It doesn't seem possible that all these different approaches can be right. Is an episiotomy beneficial to mother and baby or not? Should you be concerned about developing gestational diabetes, or should you decide not to be tested for it? Does using a monitor to continuously listen to the baby's heartbeat in labor keep the baby safer? Should you have your labor induced if you are "overdue"?

Hasn't anyone researched all of this?

Yes, someone has!

In fact, since the 1950s, literally thousands of studies have been conducted in countries all over the world, researching the risks and benefits of various tests and treatments during pregnancy and childbirth.

This is a lot of research for even the most dedicated doctor or midwife to keep up with. To make this important material available to doctors, *Effective Care in Pregnancy and Childbirth* was published in 1989 by Oxford University Press. This two-volume book provides a detailed review of the research that has been done since 1950 on care in pregnancy and childbirth. The authors, well-known obstetricians with many years of experience in both caring for pregnant women and reviewing research, began by gathering all the studies done on pregnancy and birth—everything from treatments for morning sickness to helping new babies start breastfeeding. Then they evaluated the methods that had been used to do the research and decided which studies were properly done and significant. These studies were then analyzed: if several small studies had been done on the same topic, their results were compared. The authors then made recommendations based on what the research showed. New material is constantly being reviewed and added to an updated database available on disk, called *The Cochrane Library*, published by Update Software.

The two volumes (plus a shorter paperback summary) of *Effective Care in Pregnancy and Childbirth* are extremely important, but they are difficult for pregnant women to read because they are written for physicians with a background in medical and statistical terminology. The goal of *Best Evidence* is to make this valuable information available to pregnant women and their partners.

What Is "Effective" Care?

What do we mean by "effective" care during pregnancy? Ideally, effective care would result in a healthy mother and a healthy baby. It sounds simple, but in the real world decisions about effective care can be complicated.

A normal pregnant woman is healthy, not ill. While pregnancies are usually monitored by doctors or midwives to make sure things are proceeding normally, that doesn't mean something is likely to go wrong. It's important to start with the understanding that pregnancy and birth is a process that has evolved to work very well, most of the time. In fact, even if you never had a single prenatal visit or test and gave birth at home alone, in the majority of cases you and your baby would be just fine. However, we don't recommend that approach, because there are situations where things go wrong, and a knowledgeable caregiver can make a big difference.

But because most births are normal without any intervention, it's important to consider the risks and benefits of any intervention carefully. Some procedures may only minimally improve the baby's chances of being healthy, but may greatly increase the mother's risk of complications. Some medications can reduce the pain of labor for the mother, but increase the risk of the baby having breathing problems after birth. Interventions can also affect the emotional experience of pregnancy and birth, and can affect how parents feel about themselves and their babies.

In examining the research done about pregnancy and childbirth, you should be looking for answers to three important questions:

- What kinds of interventions during pregnancy and childbirth will actually improve the outcome for women and babies? An *intervention* is anything a doctor, midwife or other caregiver might do, such as giving advice on nutrition, recommending a test or performing surgery. The *outcome* is the measurable result of that intervention for the mother and the baby. Outcomes can include effects such as more or fewer fevers, infections or injuries to the mother and more or fewer illnesses, breathing problems or need for special-care treatment in babies. An improved outcome means healthier mothers and babies.
- Are there routinely used interventions that make outcomes worse for mothers or babies?
- Are there questions we don't have answers to yet?

On some issues, research makes the choice fairly clear. Some interventions are clearly beneficial; others are clearly ineffective or even harmful. However, there are also plenty of gray areas: issues where the research doesn't come down strongly on one side or another and where there are both pluses and minuses to be considered. And there are a surprising number of situations where no good research has been done to determine whether "the way we have always done it" is effective care.

In every situation, you, as the expectant parents, are the ones who should assess the evidence available and make the decisions. Research just gives you guidelines; it doesn't make decisions for you. You are the ones who will live with the consequences and who know best what your priorities are. You are the ones who must decide what will be "effective care" for you.

Taking on this responsibility can be frightening—especially in those situations where there are no clear answers. But it is important to realize that if you simply let your caregiver make all the decisions, you are making a conscious decision to do that.

Shouldn't My Doctor Know All of This?

If all this research is available and known, why are there still routines and policies in place that clearly ignore it? This discrepancy between research-based evidence and practice happens not just in pregnancy and childbirth, but in all areas of medicine.

One reason is that practice (what doctors and hospitals actually do) sometimes lags behind the research. Doctors tend to keep on doing what they were taught in medical school, even if those procedures have since been demonstrated to be not beneficial or even to be potentially harmful. It is time-consuming and often difficult to read and evaluate all the studies that are done.

In some situations, practice leaps *ahead* of the research—as happened when electronic fetal monitors were introduced. These machines, which track the baby's heartbeat during labor, seemed, in theory, like a good idea. By the time research showed they weren't, the use of monitors was firmly established in many hospitals.

Once medical procedures are established, they are very difficult to discontinue. "The way we usually do it" becomes the standard of care in the community, even if it is not supported by research. The standard of care becomes the way in which care is measured—women expect it, and doctors expect all other doctors to do it. New techniques of unproven benefit are often introduced quickly, but when it comes to abandoning tests and procedures that have

been shown not to be helpful, inertia sets in. It's hard to admit that something you've been doing for years was useless or potentially harmful.

Also, doctors' ability to diagnose conditions is ahead of their ability to treat them. Pregnancy diabetes—more often called gestational diabetes—may be a real condition that can be diagnosed by special blood tests, and the babies of women who have pregnancy diabetes probably do have a slightly higher complication rate. But the research shows that diagnosing this condition does not mean we can do anything about it— none of the treatments for gestational diabetes has improved the complication rate at all.

Finally, medical training tends to emphasize the importance of "doing something," and so, rightly or wrongly, this has also become the usual approach to pregnancy. Even when interventions aren't likely to be helpful, "doing something" makes the caregiver (and sometimes the parents) feel better.

Physicians also have a sense that they are less likely to be sued over a complication if they have "done everything." A doctor feels more protected when a complication occurs if he or she has done a lot of tests and a Caesarean section than if he or she has sat and patiently waited for the baby to be born— even if none of those interventions could have prevented the complication.

One of the ways that standard medical practices change, though—especially in the area of pregnancy and childbirth—is to come under pressure from women who have read the research and made their own informed decisions. Your discussions with your caregiver will contribute to the ongoing improvement of prenatal care.

What This Book Can Do for You

Pregnancy and Birth: The Best Evidence will give you factual information to help you make decisions that are right for you, your baby and your family. It summarizes and explains the research, giving plenty of examples from the experiences of other women. It will also discuss how to negotiate these choices with your caregiver.

Both authors have been involved in childbirth for many years—Dr. Joyce Barrett as a family physician with a large pregnancy practice, and Teresa Pitman as a childbirth educator, doula (providing support for women in labor) and writer. To the research described in *Effective Care* we have added our own experiences, and those of women we have worked with or who have written to us about their births.

Let's imagine that right after work, Trish drops into a bookstore and buys a copy of this book. She finds out what an ultrasound is, and decides to discuss with her husband whether they want to have this done. Since midwifery is covered by her provincial health plan, Trish thinks she'll call to set up an appointment and see if this is a good choice for her. She still has lots of questions and lots of decisions to make, but now she feels she can make them based on solid information.

This book can't answer all your questions—some of them don't have answers. It can't make your decisions for you. It *can* give you a foundation of knowledge that will enable you to make your own decisions. That foundation can make you feel more confident and prepared throughout your pregnancy, labor and birth, and can help your experience be a more positive one.

The Basics of Birth

As we explain the research that has been done, we will be using many pregnancy-related medical terms. If you are already familiar with most of these, feel free to skip ahead. If not, you may find this section helpful.

The Anatomy of Pregnancy

A new baby is conceived when the sperm and the egg (or ovum) meet and fuse into a single cell, and that cell rapidly divides to form a cluster of cells. This living cluster floats to the uterus from its point of origin in the Fallopian tubes (tubes inside the mother's abdomen that lead from the ovaries, where the eggs are made, to the uterus, or womb). Once inside the uterus, the embryo (a term for the developing baby early in pregnancy) will settle into the lining of the uterus. (This lining is what comes away through the vagina during a woman's monthly menstrual period. This month the lining will stay in place, providing nourishment for the embryo, and the woman will "miss her period"—her first clue that she is pregnant.)

Some of the cells in this cluster begin to form a placenta, which will transmit oxygen and nutrients from the mother's bloodstream to the baby's. At first, the placenta consists of chorionic villae, small protrusions of cells along the wall of the uterus. When it's fully formed, the placenta will look like a large slab of beef liver with a slick and shiny membrane on one side. Out of this side emerges the umbilical cord, which attaches at the other end to the baby's abdomen. (When it dries up and falls off after the baby is born, the place where the cord was attached becomes the baby's navel.)

Pregnancy is divided into three trimesters: the first trimester is the first three months, the second trimester is the next three months, and the third trimester goes from the end of the sixth month to the baby's birth day. The number of weeks from the mother's last menstrual period is the baby's gestational age.

Within the mother's uterus, the baby (called a fetus as it continues to develop) is floating in liquid called amniotic fluid. (It's mostly water.) This fluid is contained by amniotic membranes (or just "membranes") that make up the amniotic sac or bag of waters. At the bottom of the uterus is the cervix, leading into the vagina. During pregnancy, the cervix is thick and the opening in its center is plugged with mucus. When the cervix opens and the mucus plug comes out through the vagina, it is often streaked with a little blood and is called a "bloody show."

How Labor Works

The purpose of labor is to thin out the cervix (the thinning-out process is called effacement) and pull it open (called dilation) wide enough for the baby to pass through it, into the vagina, and then out into the world. Most babies are born at full term. This means that it has been about 40 weeks since the mother's last menstrual period, give or take two weeks. A baby born earlier than 37 or 38 weeks is called preterm or premature. When the pregnancy goes on longer than 41 or 42 weeks, it is called postterm or prolonged pregnancy.

When labor starts, the uterus contracts and this pulls against the cervix. The time during which the contractions are working to open the cervix is called the first stage of labor; it can be divided into early labor, active labor and transition. Once the cervix is completely open, the baby can move down into the vagina; this is called the second stage of labor or the "pushing stage." As the baby emerges, it stretches the skin around the vagina called the perineum. Once the baby is born, the third stage of labor begins as the uterus contracts again to push the placenta out through the vagina.

When the baby is born, the midwives or physicians attending the birth will examine it and give it an Apgar score (out of 10) at one minute and five minutes after birth. To determine the score, the baby is given zero, one or two points in each of five categories: color, muscle tone, breathing, crying and response to stimulation. A low score (less than 4) means your baby probably needs extra help with breathing and coping with life outside your womb; a high score (8 to 10) tells you the baby is doing well. If your baby's score is in the middle, the midwife or nurse will keep a close eye on the baby to be sure the baby improves.

The Birth of Your Baby

Once the cervix is fully open, the baby is ready to move out of the uterus.

As the baby slips through the open cervix, the baby turns to face her mother's back.

Watch as the baby moves through the vagina by gradually lifting her head away from her chest.

Notice how the muscles of the uterus gather behind the baby, helping to ease her down and out into the world.

The baby's head crowns. As the outer vaginal tissues are stretched, the mother may experience a burning or tingling sensation.

The baby lifts her head completely away from her chest.

Watch as the baby moves her head from side to side.

This brings the baby's shoulders into position, ready to be born.

Once the baby's shoulders are born, the rest of the body will
slip out quickly.

In a matter of hours, nine months of waiting and planning
are fulfilled.

Part One

Growing a Healthy Baby

Adrienne Leong

Many women don't think much about their health until the day the pregnancy test comes back positive. You may have been smoking for several years, knowing that it wasn't the best thing for you but not worrying about it very much. Now, with a baby on the way, you're suddenly a lot more concerned. Will smoking hurt your baby? How about those beers you had before you even knew you were pregnant?

You might not have thought much about the medical care you were getting until now, either. Maybe your parents took you to a family doctor when you were a child and you just kept going to the same person as you grew up. Maybe the doctor you're seeing now was just the first name on the "available" list when you moved into your neighborhood. Now you have some big decisions to make about who should look after you and this developing baby.

As you begin to think about your pregnancy and birth, you will probably come up with even more questions. Should you sign up for prenatal classes? Where should you have your baby—at home, in a hospital or maybe in the new birthing center? What should you be eating?

Here's the best evidence about what you can do to grow a healthy baby and plan for a safe and positive birth.

Choosing a Caregiver

One of the first and most important decisions you will have to make is choosing who will provide your medical care during your pregnancy and the birth of your baby.

You should expect your caregiver to treat you with respect, to explain any procedures, tests or concerns about your pregnancy, and to be skilled and competent. Caregivers should be familiar with current research and standards. You want your caregiver to be available when you need him or her, and to have suitable arrangements made for backup care when not on call.

Those are the basics. Beyond that there is no one caregiver who will be perfect for everybody. You need to think about the kind of care you want, and then seek out the person who will provide it. Some women prefer a formal approach, while some like the camaraderie of a friendship. Some women like to discuss issues, and expect to have their ideas and feelings taken seriously; other women expect to ask questions and get answers. Some women expect their caregiver to make recommenda-tions; other women want to have options outlined, from which they will choose the one that suits them best. Some women expect emotional and psychological support from their primary caregiver; others expect to get this from their family and friends, or to be referred to another professional if they need extra help.

Susan remembers: "I knew I had found the right person when I asked if I should take vitamins, and 15 minutes later we were still talking about vitamin supplements and general nutrition." But Sandra's first appointment with the same doctor was also her last: "Everything I asked her, she would say, 'Well, that depends.' I wanted advice and she never really told me what to do." Both of these women were very happy with their choices: Susan stayed with this caregiver and Sandra found someone else she was more comfortable with.

How can women choose a caregiver who will meet their needs?

There are three kinds of caregivers currently practicing obstetrics in North America, and each has different training and often a different approach to pregnancy and birth. (In addition, doulas or labor support people may also be available in your community. Doulas do not provide medical care or catch the baby; they help provide support, encouragement, information and specific techniques for laboring women and their partners. See Chapter 18, Arriving at the Hospital.) As a pregnant woman, you need to determine which kind of care will best meet your emotional and physical needs.

Obstetricians

Obstetricians are medical doctors who have specialized in the care of pregnant women. Their medical training focuses on dealing with problems and complications; they are surgeons who perform Caesarean sections and difficult forceps deliveries. Some obstetricians do "primary care obstetrics" and will care for healthy women throughout their pregnancies. Others have a referral practice for complicated pregnancies only.

As specialists, obstetricians are very familiar with the technology used in pregnancy and birth (which has become quite complex). The routines and policies governing the care of pregnant and laboring women in hospitals are increasingly designed by obstetricians. Even though you may not go to an obstetrician for your care, it is usually obstetricians who set the rules that must be followed by family doctors and midwives in hospital.

For several reasons, a policy of having obstetricians care for woman with normal, uncomplicated pregnancies is not ideal. Obstetricians have to keep up their expertise and skills in dealing with complications, and therefore they should spend most of their time caring for "problem pregnancies." However, the vast majority of pregnancies are normal. The small percentage of complicated births in any community may not provide enough work for a full-time obstetrician. For that reason, most obstetricians also attend normal births. Unfortunately, the interventions appropriate for the complicated pregnancy may sometimes be used routinely for normal births.

There are times when an obstetrician is the best choice as your primary caregiver. If, for example, you have a health problem such as diabetes or high blood pressure before you get pregnant, an obstetrician may be the best physician to care for you during pregnancy— possibly in conjunction with another specialist. Or perhaps you discover that you are expecting triplets—again, an obstetrician may be the best person to help you with this unexpected challenge.

Pregnant women sometimes choose an obstetrician because they see these specialists as being "most qualified." The obstetrician's expertise and training, and specific interest, is generally in the area of managing pregnancy complications or problems, not in providing care for normal pregnancies. However, some individual obstetricians are very interested in working with women without any complications and in helping them have the birth they want.

Lee-Anne says, "My family doctor doesn't do births, so he referred me to an obstetrician. He very much supported my desire to have a natural, unmedicated birth. When I arrived at the hospital in early labor, he stopped by to see how I was doing, and he was very encouraging. After he examined me, he said 'Just go out and walk—go outside if you want.' So I put on my robe and my husband and I walked for hours, until the baby was almost ready to be born. That wasn't the kind of advice I expected from an obstetrician, but it worked and it suited me just fine."

Family Doctors

General practitioners or family doctors often care for pregnant women with normal pregnancies as part of their larger practice (a few family doctors choose to specialize in providing pregnancy care only). A family doctor who has cared for a woman and her family before the pregnancy is likely to have more knowledge of their particular circumstances. As Tracey comments: "Both my husband and I already knew and felt comfortable with our doctor even before I got pregnant. He knew about the problems I'd been through with the recent death of my father, and he had treated me for an earlier miscarriage that was followed by a depression. I appreciated his support and his understanding of my sometimes conflicting emotions."

The care that a family doctor can give to the majority of women whose pregnancies are not affected by any major illness or serious complication will often be more responsive to their needs than that given by specialist obstetricians. Your family doctor will handle all your health needs during the pregnancy—if you sprain your ankle or get stomach flu, these events will be handled by the same doctor with the pregnancy always in mind.

However, it is becoming increasingly common for family doctors to choose not to do obstetrics as part of their practice. The reasons for this include increased responsibility and risk of liability, poor pay for pregnancy care and more hours spent on call. They may refer pregnant women either to another family doctor who does attend births or to an obstetrician.

Pregnant women are sometimes concerned that their family doctor may be uninformed about pregnancy and birth, since it is only a small part of the doctor's overall practice. Now that more family doctors are eliminating obstetrics from their practice, those who

Finding My Caregiver—One Mother's Story

We had just moved to a new community when I found out I was pregnant with my third child. I really didn't know anyone when I came here, so it was difficult. I started my search for the doctor I wanted right away, and these are the steps I took:

- I called my old doctor to see if she happened to know anyone in this area she could recommend. No luck.
- I asked a neighbor who worked as a nurse in labor and delivery at the local hospital. She gave me a couple of names of the doctors she thought were the best. I made appointments to interview them.
- I called the childbirth educator who taught the course at the hospital and asked which doctors she would recommend. She said she didn't make recommendations.
- I went to a parent drop-in group at the parent-child center and asked about doctors. From the mothers' birth stories, I added a couple more names to my list. Some I could tell right away from the stories were wrong for me—although the mothers I talked to loved them.
- I called the local La Leche League leader and asked who her doctor was. She told me, but said he wasn't taking new patients. I wrote down his name anyway.
- I had "interview appointments" with two doctors who were on my list and taking new patients, but didn't feel comfortable with either of them. (An "interview appointment" is just what it sounds like—a time to ask questions of the doctor and

learn about his or her approach and philosophy.)

- I called the doctor the LLL leader used, and found out that he wasn't taking new patients. But a new doctor had just joined their group and she was happy to see me. I set up an appointment to meet her.
- I had a great interview and decided to have this doctor provide my care.

I didn't do this all in one week—it took a little time, but it was worth it. I'm very pleased with our new family doctor and the way she's approaching my pregnancy.

continue to attend births are generally interested in pregnancy and childbirth and make a point of keeping up to date. If problems develop that need an obstetrician's expertise, your family doctor will be able to refer you.

Midwives

Midwives are specialists in normal pregnancy and birth. If you are seeing a midwife, and complications develop with your pregnancy that the midwife does not handle, she will refer you to an obstetrician.

In some provinces midwives have full hospital privileges, so women attended by a midwife can choose either a hospital delivery or a home birth. In these communities, the midwife will provide all prenatal care as well, so the mother does not need to see a separate doctor. In other places, midwives can attend births at home, but if the woman chooses a hospital birth, a doctor must be involved as well. The midwife will generally come to the mother's home for early labor, help her decide when to go to the hospital and continue to provide support at the hospital. The doctor will then arrive and attend the birth. In that situation, the doctor may also see the mother for prenatal visits. Not all doctors are comfortable working with midwives, but your midwife will be able to give you names of doctors she has worked with in the past.

Midwives usually schedule lengthy prenatal visits, and most often the midwife you have seen for your appointments will also attend your birth. Midwives are not covered by all health plans, so you need to determine the situation where you live, and whether hiring a midwife is within your budget (most midwives have a sliding fee scale for low-income families).

Heather was living in Alberta when she became pregnant with her first child, and saw her family doctor for the first five months. Then she moved to Ottawa and sought a midwife. She was very pleased with the care her midwives provided: "Visits lasted at least an hour, were personal, comfortable and enjoyable. My midwives became like sisters or friends to my husband and me."

Research comparing midwifery (with appropriate medical backup) and traditional obstetrical care found that midwifery is associated with improved outcomes for both mother and baby. Some of these improved outcomes were "psychosocial"—women felt more supported during their pregnancies and more confident about their ability to have and care for a baby. This isn't surprising, since midwives take more time to respond to the emotional needs of the mother and family.

Midwifery also led to better physical outcomes—fewer episiotomies, fewer forceps and vacuum deliveries and fewer epidurals. This is an important benefit for both mothers and babies.

Who's Best for You?

How can you choose the best caregiver for you? Here are some factors you might consider:

1. **Where do you want to give birth?** If you have a choice of hospitals in your area, you may want to choose the hospital first and then look for a doctor or midwife who practices there. Dolores, for example, decided she wanted to have her baby at the family birthing center in a hospital not far from her home community. She says, "I chose the birthing center because of their approach to birth and the support they provide for families. When I went for a tour, I knew for sure that it was the right place for me." She was referred to the team of nurse-midwives who provide care for pregnant women and attend births at the center, and was very positive about the care she received.

   If you are planning a home birth, you will need to look for a midwife or doctor who attends home births, and you may not have many choices. (You can call your provincial midwives association; the local La Leche League may also know which doctors attend home births.)

   (See also Chapter 2, Place of Birth.)

2. **Do you have any special concerns?** Some survivors of sexual abuse, for example, feel strongly that they want to be cared for by women during pregnancy and birth, and need to choose a female caregiver who will attend their birth. For these women, a group practice where there is the possibility of being met by a male physician during labor is probably not a good option.

3. **Are there pre-existing health problems?** Diabetes, high blood pressure or other conditions, past pregnancy complications (a previous premature baby) or complications in this pregnancy (twins or triplets) might require care by a specialist.

4. **Talk to other people**. Ask everyone you know who has a baby about their experience and their caregiver. Remember that unless someone has had a really dreadful experience, most people will be positive about their doctors or midwives. Be as specific as you can in your questioning: "Did you discuss episiotomy during your pregnancy? What happened at the birth?" "My husband is concerned that a midwife will provide all the emotional support in labor, so he won't have a role to play. How did your husband find working with your midwife?" Ask about the issues that most concern you, and try to talk to as many people as possible.

5. **Who do you feel most comfortable with?** Make interview appointments (clearly designated as such when you make the booking) with all your possible choices, to see how comfortable you feel with them. Discuss your concerns with them all and see what kinds of reactions you get. (Your gut feelings are probably right!) If you are told over the phone that the practitioner doesn't do "that kind of appointment," it sends a pretty good signal that he or she is not used to being questioned.

Your Options

Your choice of caregiver will definitely be influenced by geography.

If you live in a large city, you can probably choose between a midwife, a family doctor or an obstetrician. You may base your choice on whether the practitioner attends births at home, in a birthing center or in a teaching hospital.

Women consistently prefer to see the same person during pregnancy and at the birth, or to work with a small group of caregivers and get to know all of them. This is standard practice for midwives, but is not always the case with family doctors and obstetricians. It can be stressful for women to have appointments with one doctor during pregnancy, to discuss concerns and issues and to make plans with that doctor, but to know that whoever is "on call" will show up when they go into labor.

Research supports the importance of keeping the same caregivers for pregnancy, labor and birth. Continuity of care leads to less drug use in labor, shorter labors and babies less likely to need resuscitation at birth. Parents also feel more satisfied with the care they have received.

Group practices of obstetricians or family doctors can let you know ahead of time how likely it is that your own practitioner will actually be there for your birth. Many groups arrange for you to meet all the practitioners in the group during your pregnancy, so that you will not meet a stranger when you are in labor.

However, when Margot asked her doctor if she could meet the others who shared his practice, he said that wasn't something they did. "He said that by the time I was in hard labor and the doctor showed up, I wouldn't care who it was. I knew that wasn't true! Knowing I might meet a stranger at my birth confirmed my decision to hire a labor support person (doula) to be with me and my husband throughout the whole process."

If you live in a small town or a more remote area, your choices will be much more limited. There may not be midwives in your area. Only some of the family doctors may do obstetrics, and often the obstetricians will see only women with complicated pregnancies on the

referral of their family doctor. The nearest hospital with a labor and delivery department may be far away, as the trend for small hospitals to close their obstetrics wards continues. It may be that you will see your family doctor in your own town for your pregnancy care, then be referred to a doctor in a community with a hospital two or three hours away for your labor and delivery.

If you have pre-existing health problems, it may be useful for your care to be shared by your pregnancy caregiver and your other practitioner. Christy, for example, who has been diabetic since age 10, saw both her obstetrician and her endocrinologist (diabetes specialist) during her pregnancy.

Preparing a Birth Plan

Some couples prepare a formal birth plan. This can include all the things that are important to you around your labor and birth, and what you hope your birth will be like. Some are several pages long, to cover all possible situations.

On the other hand, your birth plan might cover just one or two points that are important to you. Jacky says, "I wrote a one-line note that said, DON'T CALL ME 'DEAR'!!!" (Some women ask the nurses not to call them "Mom.") Some women write very general thoughts about their philosophy of birth; other women are very specific: "Please do not ask me at any time if I want an epidural or other painkiller. If I want it, I will ask for it."

Sometimes writing a birth plan can be a start in gathering information. Sara remembers: "I'm kind of anti-doctor, and I took this birth plan to my first appointment. It was really dogmatic—'I won't have an epidural, I won't have an episiotomy, I won't have a Caesarean section.' My doctor took me seriously and spent a lot of time talking to me about it. He pointed out a few reasonable 'what ifs'—What if I was bleeding heavily? What if my baby's heartbeat was really low and none of the things we tried improved it?—situations that made me think. I revised my plan to allow for the possibility of problems and made a point of reading more about what can happen at birth."

Mary decided her plan would be the story of her ideal birth, the one she hoped to have. She says, "Before I wrote my plan, I had a doctor and knew what hospital I was having the baby in. When I started writing, I could picture things going as I wanted up until I left for the hospital, then I couldn't imagine it after that. In my mind, I kept leaving for the hospital closer and closer to the birth. Finally, I realized that I really wanted to have my baby at home. It took a lot of doing, but I got a midwife, convinced my husband and had Samantha in my bed at home."

Birth plans can be helpful if your caregiver is in a group practice and may not be present for your birth. A copy of your birth plan can be sent to the hospital ahead of time with your pre-registration form, or you can take it with you and give it to the nurse who is admitting you. This avoids having to discuss issues with a stranger when you are in hard labor. Make sure the birth plan gets onto your chart; then it is part of the written record. Usually nurses and doctors are quite respectful of patients' written preferences; caregivers also realize that your ideas can change during labor and that your plan is not engraved in stone.

Writing a birth plan and going over it with your caregiver can sometimes be an eye-opener. Janice and Bob found that "just about everything on our birth plan our doctor said either he didn't do it that way or the hospital wouldn't allow it." Janice remembers holding Bob's hand during the discussion and feeling miserable. "The things we had written were very important to us."

Bob explains: "We wanted the baby to stay with us all the time and I was quite willing to pay for a private room so I could stay, too. Also, we didn't want our baby to have the eye drops. Neither of us has ever had any other sexual partners, so we knew our baby didn't need them. Our doctor was very pleasant but inflexible; he said that it just couldn't be as we wanted. Janice and I talked about it for hours, then changed doctors and hospitals—driving an hour farther to do it, but we were able to get agreement about everything we wanted. And it was worth it."

Your birth plan can include whatever is important to you. Sheila and Marc had requested that their own baby blankets be used to dry off the new baby, as they wanted to take these blankets home to familiarize their two dogs with the baby's smell. Sheila says, "Labor was a lot harder and more painful than I had expected. By the time the baby was actually being born, the dogs were the last thing on my mind. But the nurse had read our plan, and she had our blankets ready and a plastic bag to put them in. Afterwards, I was so pleased that they had cared enough to remember what we wanted."

There is no blank birth plan form to fill out that will suit everybody. Not everybody even wants to do one. But writing out a birth plan can help you to clarify your own priorities, reveal areas you want to learn more about and make sure that your feelings and desires are understood and respected—even when labor gets too intense for discussing issues.

Being Assertive with Your Caregiver

The teacher of the prenatal class Vijay and Jamill were attending had just finished explaining why episiotomies were rarely needed or helpful. Vijay raised his hand: "But my doctor says that almost all first-time mothers need episiotomies. Are we supposed to argue with our doctor?"

"That's my point too," said Gina, one of the pregnant women. "My doctor said I have to get the glucose tolerance test done, but you said the research doesn't support that. How can I disagree with a doctor?"

How can you become more assertive with your caregiver? This is often easier with midwives, who typically invite their clients to participate in decision making and who want them to make fully informed choices. They are often more flexible about how various aspects of pregnancy and birth will be handled.

However, some family doctors and obstetricians have developed set routines, and expect people to follow them. Most of their patients do. They may be surprised if you disagree with something they suggest, but many doctors are happy to discuss issues and concerns with you, and will respect your choices.

"My heart was pounding when I went into my doctor's office," says Marva. "I was afraid

> **The Evidence About ...**
> **CHOOSING A CAREGIVER**
>
> **Finding the right caregiver is an important, but very personal, decision. Your choices may be limited by what is available in your community. For normal pregnancies, a family physician or midwife will probably be the first choice; obstetricians focus more on complicated or problem pregnancies.**

she'd be really upset when I told her I didn't want an ultrasound. But she just said, 'Yes, you were pretty sure about your dates, weren't you?' and crossed it off on the form. It was much easier than I'd expected!"

It's true, unfortunately, that some caregivers are not very open to discussing options or to sharing decision making. In a worst-case scenario, you may decide to change to a more receptive caregiver.

2

Place of Birth: Where Will Your Baby Be Born?

As you prepare to give birth, you will decide not only who you want with you to give you support, but where you want to have your baby. How do you visualize your ideal birth? Imagine yourself in labor, and create a picture of the perfect setting. What do you see?

Elaine: "I see myself walking along the beach near our home, my feet sinking into the sand and the waves rolling in. The contractions get stronger, and we go back into the house. My midwife is there, waiting. The sunlight is coming in through the bedroom window. I get in the shower and let the water run down my back until the contractions get so strong that I want to get onto the bed."

Vicki: "I'm in the rocking chair in the birthing suite at the hospital. The curtains are drawn, the lights are dim and my tape is playing. My sister is there, talking quietly to me, and Mike is rubbing my feet between contractions. My doctor sits on the edge of the bed, reassuring me that everything is going well. I feel safe."

Some common elements that women often describe in their ideal birth settings are:

- calm, peaceful atmosphere;
- privacy—not being alone, but not feeling exposed or watched by others;
- feeling able to moan or cry out as needed;
- freedom to walk around or find a comfortable position;
- familiar, caring support people who will stay with her;
- quiet and dimly lit;
- a tub, shower or whirlpool available.

Keep your imagined ideal birth in mind as you make decisions about where you want to give birth.

Hospital Birth

Most North American women assume that they will have their babies in the hospital, just as their own mothers did.

It's hard to generalize about hospital births. Many hospitals have instituted a policy of family-centered maternity care in their birthing

Where Do You Want Your Baby to Be Born? Some Points to Consider

Birth at Home	Birthing Center	Hospital Birth
Your familiar things around you	Philosophy supports unmedicated births and minimal intervention	May be only option available in your community
Free to walk, make noises or do whatever else helps		Pain medication is usually quickly available (epidurals not always available at smaller hospitals)
Can have any support people you choose	Often have whirlpools, birthing chairs and other special equipment	
Consistent, one-to-one care from caregiver	Usually one-to-one nursing care	Emergency equipment, including operating rooms for Caesareans, is readily available
No separation from baby	Emergency equipment is readily available, if needed	
Reduced risk of infection	No separation from baby	Policies may not be the same as mother's choices (but this varies, so ask)
Unnecessary interventions are less likely	May have strict guidelines about which mothers can use the center; may have to move to regular hospital maternity ward if complications arise	Higher risk of infection
Birth can be messy—need help cleaning up		Higher risk of interventions
		Cared for by strangers
May have to move to hospital for pain medication or if complications arise		May feel inhibited about moaning or walking around

suites, and are striving to achieve a warm, home-like approach. They try to be more flexible about routines than the rest of the hospital, and to respond to the mother's needs and wishes. On the other hand, a few hospitals still routinely give enemas to women in labor, encourage laboring women to stay in bed or restrict the amount of time mother and baby can be together after birth, even though all these procedures have been shown, in research studies, to be undesirable.

Jennifer says, "When I was in labor with my first baby, I really wanted to have my sister with me for support as well as my husband. The hospital said no way, you get one support person and that is it. I felt like my husband should be there, but I know that having my sister too would have helped a lot. But it wasn't allowed."

Three years later, when Jennifer was pregnant again, she found a hospital with different policies. "When I called to ask about bringing my sister, the nurse who answered the phone told me I could bring whomever I wanted. It was up to me. I ended up bringing not only my sister, but my daughter Chelsea and my mother-in-law. It was a real family birth experience!"

Various organizations are working towards making family-centered maternity care available in all hospitals. In Canada, the Canadian Institute of Child Health in Ottawa promotes family-centered maternity care, and reports on hospitals' labor and delivery departments across the country. Health and Welfare Canada has published a book titled *Family Centred Maternity Care Guidelines*. In the United States, the Institute for Family Centered Maternity Care in Bethesda, Maryland, is active in establishing guidelines for hospital maternity care.

Even with a family-centered approach, though, most women feel that a hospital birth is a medical experience. You are given wristbands to wear just as if you were coming in for surgery; high-tech equipment is all around you; nurses you've never met before come in and out of the room where you are laboring.

In a hospital, you are also more likely to experience various interventions—and every intervention has some risk to it. If you are noisy in labor, for example—moaning or crying out—you probably will be offered medication for pain. While some women appreciate this, other women use crying or groaning to help them manage painful contractions. Other interventions, too—from fetal monitors to separation of mother and baby—are all more common in hospital births.

In some metropolitan areas, you may be able to choose between several hospitals or birthing centers. In other communities there may be only one hospital. In small towns, you may have to leave your community altogether to travel to the closest city that has a hospital that attends births.

If you have options, go for a tour of each labor and delivery unit or birthing center. It's important to ask questions about routines and any specific concerns you have, but it's also important to think about how this place makes you feel. Anne burst into tears when she saw the chilly delivery room in her local hospital, with the bright overhead light, gleaming tiles and walls lined with shiny stainless-steel equipment. She felt so unhappy at the thought of giving birth in that room that she decided to investigate home births instead.

Why Women Choose Hospital Births

You might feel more comfortable in a hospital setting. Liz, for example, already has toddler twins at home, and enjoyed the clean, efficient atmosphere of the hospital when they were born. This time, she plans to leave for the hospital with her first contractions, feeling that things will be quieter and less stressful in the hospital than in her busy, active home, where her small children are likely to want her attention when she needs to focus on laboring. She chose the local hospital both for its proximity to her home and for the peaceful setting it offers for labor.

If you have a complicated pregnancy, or a medical condition, a hospital birth will be the obvious choice for you. As governments re-evaluate the organization and funding of hospitals, they have created different levels of maternal-infant care at different hospitals. Therefore, if you have a medical problem, you may need to travel out of your home community to give birth at a hospital with the facilities you need.

Remember, too, that you can often negotiate with your hospital if some of their routines are a problem for you. It may be something as simple as wearing your own nightgown instead of a hospital gown, or wrapping your baby in the blanket you bring from home instead of one stamped with the hospital's name that helps you feel happier about your birth experience.

Home or Hospital? Martha's Story

Your plans about where your baby will be born may change during pregnancy, or even while you are in labor, depending on many things.

When Martha became pregnant with her third baby, she expected her labor would be short and intense: "My first labor took three hours start to finish. We live on a farm about 20 minutes from town. My labor just started out of the blue, fast and furious, and I could barely manage to get Curtis from the barn so we could leave for the hospital, the pains were so bad. I was only in the hospital an hour when the baby was born.

"With my next baby, the labor only took an hour. It was the same thing–it just started with long, really painful contractions right away. This time we only made it to the parking lot of the hospital–Curtis flew into Emergency yelling that I was having a baby in the car. The next thing I knew, I was on a stretcher with a crying baby on my tummy and everybody was cheering."

During Martha's third pregnancy, the local hospital closed its labor and delivery department, and Martha was told she'd need to drive an hour and a half to the hospital in the nearest city when her labor began. "Based on my past history," she says, "I knew I'd probably give birth in the car, and I didn't want that."

Martha and her husband sought out a local physician who attended home births. The more she thought about it, the more the idea of birth at home appealed to her.

Curtis, however, wasn't so sure. "The two times I had to drive Martha to the hospital in labor were the scariest times of my life. Martha was groaning and crying and I didn't know what I'd do if the baby started coming before we got to the hospital. When she had Joshua in the parking lot, there was blood all over her legs, and I was afraid she might bleed to death before I could get help. It was terrible."

While a planned home birth would avoid the drive, Curtis was afraid the doctor might not make it in time. "It would take the doctor at least an hour to get out here. And what if she was busy and we couldn't get a hold of her right away when labor started? Then it would just be me and Martha, and I was not prepared to deal with that."

Two weeks before Martha's due date, she and Curtis met with the doctor again and talked about the possibility of inducing labor in the hospital. Martha says, "I would have preferred to give birth at home, even if it meant being alone. But Curtis was dreading it, and I needed him to feel confident about what we were doing. We decided I'd go into the hospital when I hit 40 weeks and be induced."

When Martha arrived at the hospital, the doctor found her cervix already soft and starting to dilate, although Martha hadn't felt any contractions. The doctor broke the water, and within half an hour Martha was in very active labor. One hour after her induction, Martha pushed out a seven-pound baby girl.

Martha says, "It was a bit strange to go from a planned home birth to an induced labor in hospital, but it worked out well. Our situation was difficult, because my labors are so fast and we live so far from the hospital. I don't think there's any one right answer in these situations–but for us, this seemed to be the best solution."

Anna says, "I was quite happy with Callie's birth except for one thing—while I was in labor the nurses kept offering me drugs. I thought I was doing okay until one said, 'Now let me know when you want something for the pain.' I hadn't even been thinking about it until then. When the shift changed, the next nurse was even more insistent. Every time she checked the baby's heart rate, she'd ask me if I wanted anything yet. When I said no, she'd kind of shake her head, as if she thought I was making a big mistake."

When Anna arrived at the hospital to have her second baby, she told the nurse who admitted her that she did not intend to have any medication and did not want to be asked about it. "If I want drugs, I'll let you know," she told her nurse. "The care was perfect. When the labor got hard and I really started to moan, the nurse just came in and brought my husband some cream to rub on my back so my skin wouldn't get raw. When I started shivering, another nurse appeared with hot blankets to wrap around me. Finally, when I gave a real yell—I was starting to push—the nurse came in with baby blankets and put them under the warmer in the birthing room. She said, 'That sounds like we are going to see a baby soon.' That positive support was so helpful, much more than any offer of drugs would have been."

Birthing Centers

Birthing center staff are usually very respectful of the wishes of the family, and try to avoid any "protocols" around admission, labor or birth. They try not to disturb the laboring woman unnecessarily, and try to offer encouragement rather than telling the woman "how to do it." They often have a stated goal: an unmedicated birth with minimal intervention. The room is usually warm and softly lit with a selection of comfortable chairs, stools and an ordinary low bed. A large heater over the bed to keep the mother and newborn warm after the birth is a nice touch, but not essential. Typically, the family goes home within a few hours of the birth.

Kellie says, "People thought I was crazy to go the birthing center route as the center's philosophy is to go as naturally as possible (translated as 'no drugs'!). It was great. My first child was about a five-hour labor from start to finish, with the wonderful midwifery staff and, of course, my ever-supportive husband. I thoroughly enjoyed the experience and was home in four hours eating Chinese food with my new family."

Tracy also had a wonderful experience in a family birthing center. "I can't say enough about the benefits of the center and the impact it had on my birth experience. The center has two suites, which consist of a bedroom decorated with lovely linens and curtains and wallpaper, a bathroom with bidet and whirlpool tub and a sitting room with kitchen facilities, a television and a pull-out bed where my husband was able to sleep overnight."

It wasn't just the attractive setting that appealed to Tracy, though; she feels the birthing center's philosophy was even more important. "I received constant one-on-one care from a nurse trained in midwifery throughout my stay. My baby's birth was attended by my family doctor. I wore my own comfortable clothes. Once my baby was born, he did not leave my side—really my stomach or my breast—at all. He was cleaned and weighed only when I was ready to let him go for a few minutes."

Birthing centers vary widely in their policies about which pregnant women can use the center, and about drug use during labor. Some have a clear stand—no drugs—and any decision to use painkillers or drugs to speed up the labor means transfer from the birthing center to the regular labor and delivery unit of the nearby or attached hospital. Other birthing centers use injectable drugs for pain relief (for example, Demerol), but not epidurals. If you are considering using a birthing center, ask for information about their policies.

Birth at Home

The Question of Safety

Most women in North America believe that birth in a hospital is safer for their baby than birth at home. Many women who would like to deliver at home eventually dismiss the idea because they believe it is not as safe. Women often say, "I would never forgive myself if anything went wrong."

The belief that home birth is not safe is deeply ingrained in North American culture. Since 1900, the usual place of birth has changed from home to hospital. During this time period, birth has also become safer— death rates for mothers and babies have decreased steadily. These two events have often been seen as being related, but it is not a cause-and-effect relationship. The shift from home to hospital birth has not *caused* the overall improvement in infant survival.

Why do fewer mothers and babies die today than in 1900? The drop in mortality rates for *babies* has been gradual, and is almost entirely due to improved living standards, better nutrition and better overall health. Giving birth became safer for *mothers* beginning around the 1930s, and this was because of the introduction of antibiotics, safer blood transfusions, Caesarean sections for certain complications and other medical advances. These 20th-century advances have increased the safety of *both* hospital and home births.

Siblings at the Birth

Whether you are at home or in the hospital, you may want to have your older child or children present for the arrival of the newest family member. If you are considering this option, here are a few points to keep in mind:

- How does your child feel about the idea? Some children are eager to be part of the experience; others are equally firm about not being around for the birth. These feelings should be respected.
- If you are giving birth in a hospital, what are the policies about siblings being present? You may need to meet with administrative staff or even change your planned place of birth if siblings are not permitted.
- You will want to have an adult present who is responsible only for the child or children, and who is not intent on being at the birth. Even an older child who doesn't need a babysitter will need someone to be there to explain things if any problems arise.
- Movies of births can help prepare a child for the sounds and surprises of birth. You can discuss what you see on the screen and mention that you also might moan, yell or cry out, and that there might be a lot of blood. Encourage your child to discuss any concerns or fears about being at the birth.
- Be aware that children often change their minds at the last minute. The child who definitely wanted to be there might leave the room; the child who was disinterested in the whole idea might end up at his mother's side, completely enthralled as his baby sister emerges.

There is certainly no question that women who have certain complications or problems of pregnancy benefit by having treatments that are available only in the hospital. But there is no evidence that a policy of *all* women delivering in hospital is beneficial. When well-done research is analyzed, it can be shown that women having uncomplicated pregnancies do just as well at home as in the hospital. So do their babies.

That's important for women to know as they make decisions about where they want to give birth. *Birth at home for mothers with uncomplicated pregnancies attended by a skilled caregiver is as safe for mother and baby as birth in a hospital.*

This has not been an easy area to research. A randomized, controlled trial (the most reliable design for a research study, as explained in the Appendix) is not possible, as women feel strongly about where they want to give birth and are not willing to be randomly assigned.

The most useful studies have compared groups of women similar in all other respects except for place of birth. These studies have compared outcomes for planned home birth women, including those who planned to deliver at home but were transferred to hospital during labor, with a similar group of low-risk women with planned hospital births. Complicated pregnancies were excluded from both groups by screening during pregnancy. Unplanned and unattended home births were also excluded.

The conclusions: the same, very small, number of babies die in hospital as at home. The hospital groups had a higher incidence of reported fetal distress, babies who needed resuscitation at birth, babies who needed admission to the neonatal intensive care unit and higher rates of postpartum hemorrhage (bleeding by the mother after birth) than the home birth group. The incidence of interventions during labor was much lower in the home

birth group than in the hospital groups: fewer inductions, fewer artificial ruptures of membranes, fewer pain-killing drugs, fewer episiotomies, fewer forceps or vacuum deliveries.

Having a baby has risks whether the birth takes place at home or in a hospital. The goal of obstetric care is to reduce those risks as much as possible. Having a baby at home may involve choosing to accept situations that could potentially be more quickly handled in a hospital. However, choosing to have a baby in hospital also involves accepting risks—of unnecessary intervention and infection—that do not exist at home.

Why Women Choose Home Birth

The numbers of women giving birth at home remains small, but it is increasing, especially in areas where midwives are licensed and paid by health plans to attend home births.

Most women who have experienced a planned home birth become advocates. For example, Diane's first baby was born in the hospital, her second at home. She says, "I want you to know that there was nothing particularly disturbing about our eldest son's hospital birth. That is, at least, until we experienced the peacefulness of birth at home."

Wendi's first two children were born in hospital and her last one was born at home. "I have fast, violent, painful labors. With my first birth, within two hours of my admission to hospital, I was crying and screaming with the contractions. The nurse was very nice, but she kept offering me drugs because I was being so noisy. Finally I had a shot of painkiller; it made me throw up and feel really groggy. In no time at all I was feeling the urge to push anyway. I don't think anyone had expected my labor to be that fast."

With her next in-hospital labor, Wendi remembers trying not to make any noise because she felt it had been disturbing to the staff during her first labor. "I buried my face in the pillow with every contraction and just held my breath. I think it made it hurt a lot more because I felt I couldn't give in to it."

Her home birth for her third baby was "the best. By 7:30, when my husband was putting Shannon to sleep, I was moaning loudly. From 7:30 to 8:30 my contractions were two to three minutes apart and I was moaning with them. At this point, I decided to get into the Jacuzzi and sit up while pouring hot water over my belly. I was moaning and screaming. After a while, I got up to use the toilet and I felt my water break. I sat down on a mattress on the floor with my back against the couch. After a few pushes, my daughter was born. Every time I think of her birth, I remember that wonderful feeling as she came out. I had her on my chest and I checked her sex even before my midwife wiped her off."

What happens when the home birth becomes a hospital birth? Sherry's planned home birth with her first baby ended up as a hospital delivery when labor progressed very slowly. Contractions had been intense from the beginning, and after more than 28 hours, Sherry was very tired. "It was my decision to change our plans and go to the hospital. My midwives really helped by supporting my decision and pointing out how reasonable it was." An IV and epidural for the pain helped her get through the last part of the labor. Her second stage was slow because the epidural muffled her pushing urge, but with patience she had a spontaneous delivery of a healthy baby. "I feel really happy with all the decisions I made, even though it wasn't the birth I had dreamed of. The midwives really helped through the whole thing, both at home and in the hospital. I'll definitely plan on a home birth again next time, and just hope my labor goes differently."

These stories illustrate special things about birth at home. Not having to leave home avoids

What Do You Need for a Home Birth?

Your midwife or doctor will be able to provide you with a specific list of birth supplies, but you will typically need:

- waterproof, disposable pads (to sit on);
- plastic garbage bags for throwing out soiled items;
- laundry hamper lined with a plastic garbage bag (most of your laundry will be wet);
- washcloths, towels and a bowl for washing blood and fluid off you before and after the birth;
- a basin for the placenta;
- a portable lamp, a space heater if the room is cool and a heating pad for warming up receiving blankets;
- lots of receiving blankets for the baby;
- diapers and clothes to dress the baby in;
- large-sized sanitary pads (to use during labor if you are leaking fluid, as well as after the birth);
- waterproof sheet for the bed (usually you make up the bed with a clean, fitted sheet on the bottom, the waterproof sheet next and an older sheet on top. Once the baby is born, the top two layers can be stripped off, leaving a fresh clean sheet underneath for mother and baby to sleep on.);
- comfortable pyjama tops, short nightgowns or oversized T-shirts to wear during labor;
- a nursing nightgown to change into once the baby is born;
- a full tank of gas in the car and emergency phone numbers handy, just in case.

> ### *The Evidence About . . .*
> ### PLACE OF BIRTH
>
> **For low-risk mothers, giving birth at home, in a birthing center, or in a hospital are all good options.**
>
> **Where there are specific medical concerns, a hospital with appropriate facilities can reduce the risk of complications to mother and baby.**

disrupting the flow of labor. Spontaneously moving around your own house is natural and easy—there is no impediment to doing things your own way. At home, Wendi felt reassured that she could "yell all she wanted" and her midwife wouldn't mind.

For some women, giving birth at home helps remind them that it is a normal, natural process, not a medical one. Kimberley describes the birth of her daughter Skye this way: "There were no special circumstances. It was just a quiet day in our apartment with the loving support of my husband, my doula, my midwife and her partner. I labored, I pushed, I reached down and pulled out my baby, began to nurse her, and then I cried. It was simple. I did what my body told me to do and what nature intended."

3

Northern Babies: Difficult Choices

Women who live in northern Canada, far from hospitals, have to make decisions about childbirth that have never been researched by studies and that can be very difficult.

Jana, for example, recently had her sixth child. She hired a nanny to care for her older children while her husband was working so that she could travel to a southern city to give birth. "I went into labor the day I was to fly to Victoria. I had to leave at 6:30 a.m. to catch a ferry to the airport (and it was a two-hour drive to the ferry). My plane left at 10:20 a.m. I arrived in Vancouver at noon, then changed planes and flew to Victoria around 1:00 p.m. My first words to my sister were, 'I'm in labor!' to which she replied, 'Well, I guess dinner's off.' My healthy baby girl was born at 7:00 p.m."

Lois was also living in a remote northern town when she discovered she was pregnant with twins. "I was strongly advised to deliver in a large city, as facilities here would not accommodate twins. I flew to Calgary on March 1, leaving my two-year-old behind with my husband. My due date was April 1, and on March 31 I *finally* went into labor." Her twin boys were born later that day, and her husband drove 14 hours in snowy weather to pick her up. After just four days in hospital, Lois headed home with her husband and babies—a two-day trip.

Kim says her greatest fear during her pregnancy was that her baby would be born on the boat on the way into town. "We live in a remote community with no road access and our closest hospital is 22 nautical miles away. Fortunately, I had gone to town on our local freight and passenger boat on the Thursday, so I would be there for a doctor's appointment the next morning. I confidently told the crew on the boat, when they kidded me about going into labor on the trip, that I had two weeks to go." But Kim's baby decided differently. When she went into labor during the night, she had to call neighbors on an "Autotel" and ask them to please contact her husband. One neighbor hopped in his boat and traveled a mile farther down the island to wake her husband and start him traveling into town. After her son was born, Kim had to wait three days until the passenger boat sailed again to make the trip home.

Some parents decide not to make the trip into a larger community when they give birth. Daria had her baby in the tiny community hospital of her small town in northern Saskatchewan. It was a quick, unmedicated birth—and Daria commented, "Darby was born on September 18, yet she was the New Year's Baby for 1996 at our hospital!"

Rebecca says, "You must trust your own instincts and do what feels right for you, no matter what everyone else says." In her small community, she could choose either the local hospital or a hospital in the city nearly an hour away. "We decided to opt for the rural hospital, hoping we would have more individualized care. Everyone thought we were crazy. No one seemed to understand why we wouldn't want to be where the latest technology was. I am so glad we chose not to listen to those people."

Rebecca describes her birth experience as "wonderful." Hers was the only family in the hospital's small maternity wing, so they had lots of privacy and excellent care. "I felt it was the closest thing to giving birth at home."

Kim decided to have her third baby at home after the small community hospital only 45 minutes from her home closed its maternity ward. Rather than make the long trip into a larger city to give birth, she arranged to have a midwife attend her and describes her labor this way: "My labor was a mixture of hard work and fun; I used the warm bath for a while but it was so relaxing my contractions began to get irregular. So I went up to our bedroom and spent the rest of my labor beside our bed, on my knees, holding onto Bruce for support. Being in our own home made me so much more comfortable and relaxed that I occasionally laughed with the joy of it all between contractions." After her daughter

was born, Kim says, "it was heavenly to cuddle into our own bed afterwards to rest and recuperate. In the days and weeks following the birth, whenever I rested or was alone with my thoughts, happy memories of the experience made me feel all warm."

Laurie also felt it was important to trust her feelings about where to give birth. "During a perfectly normal pregnancy, I had reservations about giving birth in our small hospital in northern Ontario. My gut feeling said that this was not the place to be. So three weeks before my due date I packed a few bags, grabbed all our savings, and headed to Sault Ste. Marie (four hours south) to wait for our daughter to be born." Miranda was born five weeks later—but she arrived blue and not breathing, and had to be placed on a ventilator. A few days later she was transferred to the Hospital for Sick Children in Toronto, where she had open-heart surgery. At three weeks, Miranda had a second operation for a rare liver problem, and spent another two months in the hospital recovering before her parents were able to bring her home. Laurie is convinced that some inner mother's wisdom told her that Miranda would need this special help at birth.

Sometimes plans to head south for the birth are changed when the baby decides to make an early arrival. Tracey had planned to leave her small community in northern Ontario and have her baby in Toronto, where she had relatives. However, three weeks before her expected due date, Tracey's water broke. She headed for her community hospital, only to find that her family doctor was away on holidays and the only other doctor in town who delivered babies was off on a shopping trip. Tracey was having contractions at this point, and the doctor in charge decided to send her, strapped onto a stretcher, by helicopter to Thunder Bay, the closest city. Tracey remembers: "My husband was not allowed on the helicopter and had to drive the four-hour trip to Thunder Bay. Fortunately, he made the trip safely and I delivered a healthy baby girl that evening. All we faced now was getting her home in the middle of winter."

Families in the more remote communities of northern Canada have a number of decisions to make that families in other parts of Canada may never consider. If they decide to travel south before the expected arrival time of the baby, the expenses of staying in the city can quickly mount up, especially if there are no friends or family with a handy spare room.

Inducing labor looks far more appealing when every day you wait for labor to begin means more money paid out for food and hotel bills, as well as another day separated from your older children and your partner. Some mothers have described feeling depressed and lonely as they waited out their pregnancies "in the company of strangers." Those who had family to stay with were more positive about the experience, but it was still difficult to be away from their partners.

If the mother decides to stay in her home community to give birth, she may have a very positive experience. However, if she or the baby needs extra care, it may mean a sudden, traumatic trip by plane or helicopter to a larger hospital.

There is no right decision in these situations. Each family has to weigh the resources available in their community and their own feelings to make a plan that is right for them.

4

Prenatal Classes: Do They Help?

Forty years ago, there were very few prenatal classes. Pregnant women gathered information from their sisters and friends, from their mothers and from their medical caregivers. Often they were simply told not to worry—after all, the doctor would take care of everything.

The earliest prenatal classes were like present-day school health classes: teaching women about their bodies and the changes that occur during pregnancy. Women were told that the doctor and nurses would tell them what to do during labor and birth.

In the 1960s, prenatal class teachers focused on avoiding the painkillers that were widely used at the time during labor. These classes emphasized breathing patterns to help women "stay in control" and not make noises during contractions. These lessons were important because if the laboring woman showed signs of pain or distress, the hospital staff were likely to urge her to take medication.

Through the 1970s and 1980s, prenatal classes gave more information to pregnant women and their partners. Women learned about nutrition, alcohol consumption and smoking in pregnancy, the growth of the fetus and the different stages of labor. The classes also taught that many hospital policies in place at the time were not necessary—you don't need to be shaved, you don't need an enema, you don't need an intravenous. Avoidance of pain medication during labor was accepted as a good thing, and pain-relieving techniques such as massage and "patterned breathing" were encouraged. Some classes concentrated on vaginal birth after Caesarean section (VBAC) in the days when it was much less accepted by the medical community than it is now. Prenatal classes became a force for change from rigid hospital birthing policies to the adoption of family-centered maternity care.

At present, most prenatal classes have some things in common. They provide information about pregnancy, fetal development and stages of labor. They teach techniques such as position change, massage and breathing patterns to help cope with labor pain. Most discuss common interventions in labor, including those for pain relief. Care of the new baby, and changing relationships between the couple, any older children and the new baby, are discussed. Beyond those basics, though, there are a variety of special prenatal classes that may be available in your community. Each will have a different focus and approach.

Steffi attended a prenatal class for single teen mothers. "We only had one class about the birth, and that was mostly to tell us what to expect at the hospital. I liked the hospital tour; it helps to see the rooms before you actually go. We had a lot of stuff about nutrition, getting welfare, finding a place to live and birth control."

Jeanine's prenatal classes were taught by an independent childbirth educator at the local Y. "I have to confess that Jack didn't like them much, because after each class I'd go back and argue with our doctor. A lot of the things the teacher talked about were different than what our doctor usually did. Jack thought the teacher was pretty much against the whole medical system. But it opened my eyes. I found out there were other ways of doing things."

She adds: "We did do some breathing and relaxation stuff, too, and we practiced quite a bit. When I was in labor, what I had learned in the classes helped me a lot. I had a lot of back pain in labor, but I knew from the classes that it was pretty common, and we'd learned some things that helped, like having Jack press hard on my back."

Manuela's classes were taught by the nurses at the hospital. "We learned about what happens during labor and birth. The nurses were able to show us how the fetal monitor works and they brought in the vacuum extractor and

the forceps, so we had a chance to get familiar with everything. I liked knowing what was available for pain, and what would happen to me in labor."

Sherry's classes were taught by her midwife. "We'd actually discussed most of the issues during my prenatal visits, so I didn't learn all that much. The best parts were watching the videos of birth, and getting to know other pregnant couples who were going through the same things we were. We talked a lot about our fears, our feelings about becoming parents, our relationships."

No class can cover everything in detail. Lee Ann says, "My prenatal classes had mentioned that one in five moms don't deliver naturally, but instead of educating us on Caesareans, the class focused on the four moms who would deliver vaginally. But there we were—I was Mom Number Five who needed a Caesarean."

Some classes teach a wide variety of labor skills that include relaxation techniques, breathing patterns, distraction, comfort measures, movements, etc. Others cover these briefly but focus more on the medications (such as narcotics and epidurals) available for pain relief. Some place a lot of emphasis on teaching labor support skills to the woman's labor partner, while others barely discuss the partner's role.

Classes vary in their overall attitude towards labor and birth. In some classes, labor is approached as something that women are taught to manage through breathing and relaxation techniques. As the coach, the father is to remind the mother what to do. In other classes, the approach is that labor is something that women instinctively know how to do. The other people present are not seen as coaches, but as a source of support. Some classes treat birth as a normal event with profound spiritual and emo-

Choosing a Prenatal Class

What should you be looking for when you choose your prenatal classes?

In a small community, you may not have much choice; there may only be one set of classes available. Then it becomes particularly important to supplement the classes with outside reading and discussions with your caregiver and your friends.

If you do have a choice of classes, here are some points you might consider:

- Ask your caregiver. Your doctor or midwife will know what classes are available and may feel that one is preferable.
- Do you have some special circumstances that might point you towards a particular class? Single mothers, for example, sometimes feel more comfortable in a class specifically for single parents. Some communities offer separate classes for couples who are expecting twins or other multiples, for those planning a vaginal birth after a previous Caesarean section, for those planning a home birth or for survivors of sexual abuse.

  If you are considering one of these special classes, discuss the course outline with the teacher to be sure it meets your needs. Not all single mothers, for example, need information on applying for welfare and public housing, and some may prefer a class where the emphasis is on preparing to give birth.

- What books does the class teacher recommend for further reading? Checking out the book list will help you to identify the teacher's philosophy and approach so that you can decide if it fits with yours.
- What do new parents say about the classes they attended? When people tell you the classes they attended were "great" and "wonderful," don't just accept that at face value. What is great for one person might be boring and frustrating for another. Ask them what they found helpful, what they learned that was useful during labor, anything they wished had been included in the class but wasn't. This will give you information that will help you to decide if the class is right for you.

Even with a prenatal class that matches your needs and philosophy, don't forget the other resources available to you: books, magazines, videos (your public library probably has a number of videos on childbirth that you can borrow) and more.

If you have access to the Internet, there are newsgroups, bulletin boards and chat lines on all aspects of pregnancy, childbirth and parenting where people share experiences and offer answers to questions.

tional aspects. These classes are likely to encourage questioning of medical routines and interventions. Other classes encourage cooperation with medical personnel and acceptance of a more technological approach.

The Effects of Prenatal Classes

Because of these wide variations, it is very difficult to research any benefits or disadvantages of prenatal classes. As well, women who choose to take prenatal classes may be inherently different than those who don't, so differ-

Preparing for Birth: What Are Your Options?

Depending on where you live, you may have many choices in prenatal education or only a few. Some possibilities:

- Preparation for home birth (may be taught by your midwife)
- International Childbirth Education Association classes (independent class taught by certified instructors)
- Preparation for Caesarean section classes
- Early pregnancy classes (focus on nutrition, exercise and healthy pregnancy)
- VBAC classes
- Hospital-based classes taught by nurses
- Single parent or teen mother classes
- Classes for parents expecting twins or multiples
- Refresher classes for people expecting a second or later baby
- Bradley Method classes (husband-coached childbirth)
- Weekend all-day workshop classes (for people who find it difficult to attend evening classes on a regular basis)
- Breastfeeding preparation (often offered as an "extra" class)

ent outcomes in the two groups may be due to factors other than the classes.

However, studies have been done, and one clear difference has emerged: women who have attended prenatal classes use significantly less pain medication during labor than those who have not attended any classes. This is a very important positive outcome, because all of the pain medications currently available can cause side effects in the mother and risks for the baby.

Concern has been expressed that prenatal classes create expectations of a "natural birth" that is impossible for some women, and that these women consequently either suffer unnecessary pain in labor or suffer feelings of guilt and failure if they decide to ask for pain medication. This possibility—that classes may do harm—has not been evaluated by research in any systematic way.

When prenatal classes make women aware of options and choices and pass along accurate information, they can be a vital agent for change. It was because many women learned about their choices in prenatal classes that hospitals began to change their policies around allowing labor support people, changing positions for birth, walking during labor, etc.

As Jeanine says, "Talking to the other women in my prenatal classes was very enlightening. At my hospital, the rule was that every woman in labor got an IV. Well, if that's medically necessary, how come at Linda's hospital it was *not* part of the routine? Why did babies at my hospital go to the nursery for eight hours after birth for observation, while the babies at Daria's hospital stayed with their mothers? If I hadn't been to the classes, I wouldn't even have known about those possibilities."

When parents like Jeanine talk to their doctors and write letters to their hospitals asking for changes, they can have a real and significant influence on the practice of obstetrics in their community.

Prenatal classes can also have the opposite effect. Ask Manuela if anyone questioned the nurses who taught her class, and she says, "Yes, a couple of people asked about stuff they'd read or heard about. But the nurses explained that some of these books are really radical and the people who write them aren't nurses or doctors and don't really know what they're writing about. On the other hand, there are hundreds of babies born at this hospital every year, so they obviously know what they're doing." This kind of class discourages questioning of medical routines and will probably reduce the level of change at that hospital.

The Evidence About...
PRENATAL CLASSES

Attending prenatal classes is likely to reduce your need for pain medication during labor.

The classes will also provide you with information and opportunities to meet other expectant parents.

5

Nutrition and Exercise

Tara is just out of her teens, single—which in her case means she doesn't have much money—and pregnant. For the past few years, because she's very concerned about staying slim, she's been alternately dieting (eating nothing but celery and carrot sticks for a week) and bingeing (on french fries and burgers) when her willpower gives out. Now she's pregnant, and her main concern is not gaining too much weight so she'll still fit into her jeans after the baby is born. She does, however, want her baby to be healthy.

Selene is also pregnant. She's been a vegetarian for most of her life, enjoys planning and preparing meals, and is very interested in nutrition. She also takes a number of herbal supplements and vitamins, and wonders if these are safe during pregnancy.

Marta doesn't think much about food. Her husband jokes that the oven in their apartment has never been turned on! Because he and Marta are both very busy at work, they eat almost all their meals out—and because they're usually in a hurry, it's often at "fast food" restaurants. Marta doesn't see that changing much now that she's pregnant, but she's worried about how this diet will affect the baby.

Connie's expecting her sixth child and her oldest is not yet 10. She feels more tired this time than during her previous pregnancies, but doesn't have much time, energy or money to worry about nutrition. Her focus is on preparing meals her children will eat and that she can afford, so she tends to serve a lot of pasta, rice and potatoes. She wonders whether this is good enough to grow a healthy baby.

Four pregnant women, each with very different nutritional histories, different lifestyles and incomes and different concerns about nutrition during pregnancy. In fact, every pregnant woman's nutritional status will be unique, and that's what makes it impossible to say that there is one "ideal diet" for every pregnant woman.

What do we know about nutrition during pregnancy? The truth is, not a lot. There are so many possible variables that this is a very challenging area to research. Most of the studies that have been done focus on supplementation of the diet, because this is easier to measure than what people actually eat.

Pregnancy Supplements: The Daily Dose of Vitamins and Minerals

Although multivitamin supplements for pregnant women have been recommended by doctors for years, the actual required amounts of each vitamin or mineral have not been determined by research in most cases.

Folic Acid

The supplement that research has found to be most helpful during pregnancy is folic acid. Taking 0.8 mg per day of folic acid, beginning *before* pregnancy occurs and continuing through the first trimester, significantly reduces the risk of the baby having neural tube defects, either anencephaly or spina bifida. Anencephaly means the baby develops without a brain; these babies are either stillborn or die shortly after birth. Spina bifida is an abnormality of the spinal cord that can cause paralysis of the legs and lack of bladder and bowel control. Without folic acid supplements, the risk of a woman having a baby with a neural tube defect is 1 to 2 per 1000. Although this defect is already rare, because the disease is so severe, the reduction in risk with folic acid is important.

Women who have already had a baby with a neural tube defect have a higher risk of having another one in a subsequent pregnancy. They can reduce this risk by two-thirds by taking a higher dose—4 mg per day—of folic acid from before pregnancy until the end of the first trimester.

It's easy to take folic acid supplements once pregnancy is known, but half of all pregnancies are unplanned. The folic acid must be taken before conception and during the early weeks of pregnancy for the risk of neural tube defects to be reduced. To get an adequate amount of folic acid from food alone, the diet must include meat, milk, orange vegetables and fruits, dark green vegetables and legumes.

Iron

Although multivitamin supplements for pregnant women all contain iron, taking extra iron during pregnancy isn't supported by the research.

It is normal for the amount of iron in a woman's blood to drop during pregnancy, but this does not mean it is a problem that needs to be corrected. In fact, the lower iron levels indicate that the mother now has a higher blood volume, something that is normal and desirable in pregnancy.

Iron supplements have been routinely given to pregnant women for many years, but no benefits have been detected. The supplements do raise the measured level of iron in the mother's blood, but this does not improve the overall outcome for either the mother or the baby. None of the studies indicate improvement in incidence of low birth weight babies, high blood pressure in pregnancy, excessive bleeding after delivery or stillbirth. This means that routine iron supplementation is at least wasteful, and can give a woman the mistaken impression that her nutrition is not adequate or that her body is not working properly.

Women do not feel better for having their hemoglobin (the measure of iron-containing red cells in the blood) made higher with iron supplements. In fact, iron supplements frequently contribute to constipation. Of more concern, two recent studies found that iron supplementation resulted in an increase in the number of babies born prematurely or with low birth weight.

Women who were anemic because of iron deficiency before they became pregnant *should* receive iron supplements. However, iron supplements for all pregnant women are not recommended.

Vitamin D

Vitamin D is mainly obtained from exposure to the sun and from certain foods (such as milk). Women who don't drink milk or eat cheese and who have very little exposure to the sun may become vitamin D deficient. These women's babies will have less risk of low blood calcium at birth (which makes the baby irritable) if their mother's diet is supplemented with Vitamin D during pregnancy.

Vitamin B$_6$

Vitamin B$_6$ supplements may protect mothers against dental decay when taken during pregnancy, but no other benefits have been demonstrated.

Magnesium

Magnesium supplements were found in some studies to reduce the number of premature births and the number of low birth weight babies, but these studies were too small and too poorly done to allow any reliable conclusions.

The amounts that should be taken of each of these vitamins and minerals, other than folic acid, have not been established. If you feel that your diet needs to be supplemented (for example, if you are exposed to very little sunlight and are concerned about your levels of vitamin D), you should consult with a dietitian or nutritionist about the amounts of particular nutrients that would be appropriate for your situation.

Diets to Prevent Allergies

Enza comes from a family with a history of allergies. She herself suffers from hay fever, asthma and allergies to seafood and strawberries. Her first baby has eczema and asthma, and is allergic to milk.

When Enza became pregnant again, she decided to try avoiding potentially allergenic foods to see if this would prevent allergies in her new baby. "I didn't drink milk or have any dairy products," she says, "and I stayed away from citrus fruits and nuts."

When people asked Enza about getting enough calcium, she pointed out that in many parts of the world most adults do not drink milk or eat dairy products. Despite this, they continue to have healthy babies. Calcium is present in many foods, including green leafy vegetables, canned salmon (with bones included) and almonds. Calcium supplements are also available for those who worry that their diet is not adequate.

This baby, however, also has some allergies—but not to milk. "I can't really tell if the special diet made a difference," Enza says, "but I think it may have prevented the milk allergy."

Did it? Studies suggest that even on these special diets, women with a family history of allergies are still more likely to have babies with allergies. More research needs to be done. It is difficult and unreasonably expensive for pregnant women to plan nutritious meals when entire food groups are excluded or many foods are eliminated, if there is no evidence their babies will benefit.

Herbal Supplements: All-Natural Doesn't Always Mean Safe

Caution is recommended in taking herbal supplements. Some herbs can be dangerous during pregnancy, even though they are "natural." The labeling on herbal supplements is sometimes incomplete, so you may not know exactly what you are taking. Make sure you know all the ingredients of any herbal teas or other natural supplements you are considering, and check with your midwife or doctor before taking any herbal supplements while you are pregnant.

Nutritional Attempts to Prevent Pre-eclampsia

We've already pointed out that folic acid supplements can contribute significantly to reducing spina bifida, a serious birth defect. Researchers and doctors have searched for similar nutritional approaches to other pregnancy complications—in particular, pre-eclampsia (formerly called toxemia).

Pre-eclampsia (see Chapter 12, Hypertension and Pre-eclampsia) is a disease in which the mother's blood pressure goes up, protein is found in her urine and she becomes swollen from retained fluids. This is a serious condition for both mother and baby.

In the past, many doctors believed that minimizing weight gain in pregnancy would prevent pre-eclampsia. While a certain amount of weight gain was "permitted," the woman who managed to gain less was praised. Unfortunately, research shows that restricting weight gain during pregnancy does not prevent pre-eclampsia. Pregnant women have also been told not to eat salt, because of the belief that high salt intake might be related to the high blood pressure seen in pre-eclampsia. Again, research shows no benefits to reducing (or increasing) salt intake.

Some nutritionists have suggested that higher protein intake during pregnancy could reduce pre-eclampsia rates, but this has not been borne out by research. Calcium supplements have also been considered as a possible preventive measure, but a recently published large study found no benefit to calcium supplementation in preventing high blood pressure or pre-eclampsia.

So far, we have not discovered any modifications of diet and nutrition (or any non-nutrition approaches, either) that will prevent pre-eclampsia. However, you may still hear recommendations to avoid salt or eat more protein, particularly from people who had babies 15 or 20 years ago.

Weight Gain: How Big Will That Belly Grow?

Although it is now clear that restricting weight gain will not prevent pre-eclampsia, checking the mother's weight continues to be a part of most prenatal visits. In some cases, this becomes a source of significant—and unnecessary—stress for the mother.

In the past, women were usually urged to limit their weight gain. Doctors believed that gaining the least weight possible would produce a smaller baby who would be easier to deliver. It is true that severe dietary restrictions can cause smaller babies, but this is not a positive thing. In famine conditions—when no one, including pregnant women, gets enough to eat—the average weight of babies can drop by almost a pound. There is no evidence that this produces an easier birth for the mother, and there is definite evidence that smaller-than-average babies are more likely to have health problems after birth.

More recently, a higher weight gain of 25 to 35 pounds (and more for multiple preg-

Nutrition and Exercise   45

The Pregnant Woman and the Food Police

Throughout history and around the world, women have always been warned about the foods they must eat or should not eat during pregnancy. Here are just a few examples:

- English mothers were warned not to eat strawberries, or the baby would be born with a strawberry birthmark.
- Mothers in Malta were told that if they craved a certain food they must eat it, or the baby would be born with a handicap. At family gatherings, pregnant women always chose their food first and were encouraged to choose the foods they craved.
- Mothers in Siberia were advised not to eat eggs during pregnancy, or their babies would be born deaf.
- The pregnant Thai woman was told not to eat hot chili peppers, which would give her baby a "hot temper," but instead to eat cool

foods such as bananas to create a calm baby.
- In northern India, mothers are traditionally given yak's milk to drink during pregnancy to make the baby strong and fortunate. In other parts of India, honey and butter are eaten during pregnancy to ensure the baby's well-being.
- European Gypsy women believed that eating crayfish during pregnancy would cause a more painful and difficult labor.
- Women in the East Indies believed they needed to eat a special seafood soup in the days after delivery to have a good supply of breast milk.

Not much different, perhaps, than the warnings North American women were given in recent years to avoid salt or to eat large amounts of protein during pregnancy.

nancy) has been encouraged. This is probably a positive move away from the earlier emphasis on restricting weight, but may not allow enough for the variations in normal women. As Margaret found, "I am only 5'3" and usually weigh about 100 pounds. I felt like I was stuffing myself all the time trying to gain enough weight, and I'd only managed 22 pounds by the end of my pregnancy. My doctor kept nagging me to eat more, but it was impossible." Margaret's baby girl weighed a healthy 7 lbs. 6 oz. when she was born.

Overweight women are frequently told to restrict their weight gain during pregnancy. Debbie, who weighed 200 pounds pre-pregnancy, was told to gain no more than 15 pounds during her first pregnancy;

when she hit 14 pounds at six months, she knew she was in trouble. "I wouldn't eat anything at all the day before my doctor's appointment," she says. "But then I'd have to do the same thing the next month, and it was pretty stressful." In the end, Debbie gained 26 pounds, dreaded every doctor's appointment and had an 8 lb. 8 oz. healthy baby boy.

Some studies have been done with overweight women who were placed on low-calorie diets during pregnancy, but these have not shown any clear effects on the size of the baby or the health of the mother.

"There is no justification for allowing pregnant women to go hungry, or for imposing dietary restrictions upon them," write the authors of *Effective Care in Pregnancy and*

Childbirth. In other words, it is important to pay attention to your appetite, and not to be ruled by the numbers on the bathroom scale at home or in your doctor's office.

So What Should I Eat?

If you've wondered why your caregiver tends to respond to this question with a muttered "just eat a balanced diet," now you know. Nutrition during pregnancy has not been widely researched, even though it is of considerable concern and interest to most pregnant women.

Some of the research done on nutrition is a little discouraging. Supplementing the diet of malnourished women with extra protein alone actually resulted in a higher incidence of small babies. When researchers tried to supplement the diets of malnourished women with more calories balanced in fat, carbohydrate and protein, the babies born were still very small. This suggests that it takes more than nine months to repair the effects of many years of malnutrition. It may be that the food you eat *before* you conceive is as important as the food you eat during pregnancy.

However, good nutrition is known to make an important contribution to overall health, and it seems reasonable to suppose that it plays a role in healthy pregnancy, too. A diet that includes plenty of whole grains, fruits and vegetables, and moderate amounts of dairy products, meats and/or other protein foods seems likely to be the best approach, as it is for non-pregnant women. Including a wide variety of foods from each food group, and eating foods with minimal processing, will help to ensure that you are getting all the important nutrients. A vegetarian diet with adequate protein is perfectly good nutrition during pregnancy. Women with lactose intolerance who avoid milk can continue to avoid dairy products during pregnancy, but should include adequate amounts of other foods containing calcium.

If you are concerned about eating appropriately during pregnancy, especially if you have a past history of eating disorders or other nutritional problems, ask your caregiver to refer you to a dietitian or nutritionist who can evaluate your nutrition, height and weight, and lifestyle to help you find an affordable and healthy eating plan.

Working Out: Exercise During Pregnancy

Good research on exercise in pregnancy is difficult to do. Because women who exercise are often different in other ways from women who don't exercise, it is hard to make proper comparisons. Most of the available research looks at women who identify themselves as exercising regularly and compares them to the general population of pregnant women. The conclusions from these studies are:

- Exercise in pregnancy is a good thing. It's good to continue exercising if you have always done it, and it's good to start during pregnancy even if you haven't exercised before.
- Exercise in pregnancy helps mothers to sleep better and feel less depressed. Women who exercise have faster labors, fewer inductions, fewer forceps deliveries and fewer Caesarean sections.
- Exercise does not cause miscarriage.
- Exercise is associated with uterine contractions, but is not associated with an increased chance of premature birth.

You may want to try out different activities to stay comfortable while you are pregnant. If

The Evidence About...
NUTRITION AND EXERCISE

Folic acid supplements taken before conception and during the first trimester can reduce the risk of neural tube defects in the baby.

Iron supplements for all pregnant women are not recommended.

Vitamin D may be helpful in a few situations, and calcium and magnesium supplements need further research.

Pre-eclampsia cannot be prevented by any known nutritional strategies.

Weight gain during pregnancy should not be restricted.

Nutrition during pregnancy has not been widely researched. Women with specific concerns or problems should consult a dietitian or nutrition expert.

With appropriate safety precautions, exercise in pregnancy is beneficial for the mother and safe for the baby.

running makes you feel like you have to urinate every time the baby bounces against your bladder, try walking instead, or biking, or swimming.

Because your body changes during pregnancy, three safety precautions are recommended:

1. Warm up thoroughly before you exercise. This is important because your ligaments are more lax, your joints are looser than normal and your abdominal and back muscles are stretched.

2. Avoid exercising to the point of breathlessness, or until your heart rate is over 100 to 120 beats per minute. Intense exercise will divert the blood and oxygen to the muscles and away from the baby. For the well-conditioned athlete, this will mean exercising at a lower level than usual.

3. In the last trimester, you should also avoid floor exercises where you are lying on your back, as this position reduces the blood flow to your uterus and your baby.

6

Lifestyle Risks: Smoking, Drinking and Drugs

When a Manitoba woman, pregnant with her fourth child, was brought to court by the child welfare system to force her to get treatment for her solvent-sniffing addiction, the country's attention was drawn in a very dramatic way to the issue of drugs during pregnancy. This mother's previous three children were already in the care of the Children's Aid Society and showed clear evidence of damage due to their mother's drug use during her pregnancies. In the commentary on this case, it was pointed out that many women smoke cigarettes or consume alcohol in amounts that put their babies at increased risk. Should these women, as well, be forced into treatment programs?

The Manitoba court decided that the pregnant woman could not be legally required to undergo treatment for her addiction. The Supreme Court of Canada upheld this opinion: "Nobody has the legal right to interfere with a pregnant woman whose behavior threatens her fetus." This judgment supports women's right to make their own decisions, including harmful ones. It does nothing to settle society's responsibility to that fetus. Another statement from the Supreme Court decision rings very true from the medical point of view: "The mother and her fetus are one."

The research in some areas is quite clear. "Recreational" drugs—including tobacco, alcohol and illegal drugs from glue-sniffing to crack cocaine—put the developing fetus at risk.

Smoking

Smoking leads to a slightly increased risk of miscarriage, an increased risk of accidental separation of the placenta, reduced birth weight and an increased risk of Sudden Infant Death Syndrome (SIDS, sometimes called "crib death") after the baby is born. What isn't clear is how to best help pregnant women who are addicted to cigarettes. Simply telling women to stop smoking does not help them with their addiction, and hearing lectures about the dangers of smoking during pregnancy can make women feel guilty and inadequate. We do not know if feeling stressed and anxious harms pregnancies or affects the mother's subsequent relationship with her baby. But the stress of knowing she is potentially causing problems for her baby may actually increase the tobacco-addicted woman's desire to smoke—10 percent of women who smoke actually smoke *more* when they are pregnant.

For other women, pregnancy can provide the motivation they've been looking for to stop smoking. Kim says, "I'd been talking about quitting for years. When I got pregnant, I decided this was the time. One of my worries had been that I would gain weight if I quit smoking, so pregnancy was a good time to quit—I was gaining weight anyway!"

The ideal situation would be to give up tobacco before the baby is conceived, but this isn't always possible. For pregnant smokers, referral to the Lung Association or the local public health department for smoking cessation courses is useful. Specific behavioral strategies are much more likely to help women to stop smoking than is simple advice. There are a variety of programs currently available for those who want to stop smoking, even if you have to check out a couple before you find one that suits you. Having your partner quit with you not only gives you some support while you quit, but a non-smoking household is healthier for the baby after birth (having parents who smoke is a significant risk factor in SIDS and in lung infections and asthma in infants).

If the mother can't quit smoking altogether, it is useful to cut down. The harm from cigarettes seems to be "dose related," and although research has not determined a safe lower level, it appears that the less smoked the better.

Alcohol

Alcohol is the most commonly used recreational drug in the world. There is no evidence to suggest that an occasional drink is harmful to the fetus. Rather, harm appears to be caused more by steady, regular consumption or heavy binges during pregnancy.

Fetal Alcohol Syndrome is a condition seen in some babies whose mothers have been steady drinkers throughout pregnancy (averaging two drinks per day or more), although some affected babies have been born to mothers who binged heavily on only a few occasions. Babies with FAS usually have small, abnormally shaped heads and are developmentally delayed. Large amounts of alcohol during early pregnancy seem to be most likely to cause problems for the fetus—and this is a concern, because about 50 percent of pregnancies are unplanned and many women don't realize they are pregnant in the early weeks. However, you shouldn't be concerned about those two glasses of wine you had when your period was just a couple of days overdue.

Fetal Alcohol Effect is a less obvious complication of alcohol exposure during pregnancy. The infant has no physical signs at birth, but has developmental problems during childhood. Children with Fetal Alcohol Effect have trouble connecting cause and effect, and often act on impulse because they don't think ahead.

Research hasn't determined if regular low levels of alcohol consumption are safe, or if it is safe for the fetus when the mother doesn't drink all week but has several drinks on Friday and Saturday nights.

Like addiction to cigarettes, alcohol addiction is a complicated disease that is difficult to treat. The information available about Fetal Alcohol Syndrome tends to worry women who are light or infrequent drinkers during pregnancy, even though their babies are not likely to be at risk. However, simply being told that heavy drinking may affect the baby isn't likely to help a woman who is addicted to alcohol.

Illegal Drugs

The effects of illegal drugs depend on the amount and frequency of drug use, and on the particular drugs involved. Babies born to mothers who are addicted to heroin or cocaine are also born addicted to the drug from their exposure to it in the uterus. Addicted babies go through withdrawal symptoms after birth, and many have developmental delays and health problems as they grow up. As with cigarettes and alcohol, information only about the risks seems to have minimal effect on drug usage during pregnancy in women who are already using drugs. These women need a concrete program for drug withdrawal.

Prescription and Over-the-Counter Drugs

The rule with any medication you might take during pregnancy is caution.

Some prescription drugs have been studied and are felt to be safe during pregnancy—for example, some antibiotics, high blood pressure medicine, anti-nausea pills and painkillers.

Many drugs have not been specifically researched for safety for the developing baby; they might be safe, we just don't know for sure. These are usually labeled: "Safety in pregnancy not established; weigh the potential benefits against the possible hazards to the fetus." This

is good advice—if you can manage without them, don't take them.

Some drugs are thought to be dangerous for the developing fetus, usually because animal studies have demonstrated teratogenicity (this means the drug causes fetal abnormalities). Tragically, some drugs (such as thalidomide) are known to be teratogenic to humans because they were given to pregnant women before the danger was known.

Whenever you are given a prescription, remind the doctor that you are pregnant. If you have forgotten to mention it to the doctor, you can ask the pharmacist to check the drug's safety for you before you fill the prescription. Most diseases have more than one possible treatment. If one drug is not safe during pregnancy, another may be.

Filomena developed pneumonia during her second pregnancy. "I was really sick, I felt terrible. But it wasn't easy to find the right medication, because I was allergic to one antibiotic and the other one the doctor recommended wasn't safe during pregnancy. The one I ended up with was probably the least effective. I needed to stay in bed and rest much longer than I might have with a different antibiotic, but eventually the pneumonia cleared up—and I felt my baby was safe."

Caution is also recommended if you are considering herbal remedies. The fact that these medications are from natural sources does not necessarily mean they are safe for the baby. Check with your midwife, naturopath or physician before taking any herbs, including herbal teas.

Drugs are a very common part of our lives, and many of us consume tobacco, alcohol, aspirin, allergy pills and more without thinking about their possible risks.

The Evidence About...
SMOKING, DRINKING AND DRUGS DURING PREGNANCY

Smoking, drinking and drugs (both recreational and prescription) can harm the fetus.

We have to use this knowledge to develop helpful strategies for addicted women; simple advice to stop smoking, drinking or taking drugs is not useful. Women who are concerned about their use of these substances are encouraged to seek out treatment programs that will give them practical strategies and ongoing support for quitting.

Knowledge about the harmful effects of alcohol has raised unnecessary fear in women who have had an occasional drink in early pregnancy.

The rapidly growing fetus is very sensitive to many of the chemicals we take in, and pregnant women need to be aware and cautious.

For more information about specific drugs and their safety during pregnancy, you can contact the Motherisk phone line at the Hospital for Sick Children in Toronto at 416-813-6780. Pauline says, "Please tell mothers about the Motherisk number. The person who spoke to me was so helpful, and I felt very reassured that the medication my doctor was recommending was safe."

Part Two

Tests During Pregnancy

TCL/Masterfile

Your baby may be hidden from view within your belly, but you can take a peek inside with some of the new tests and technologies. Is this a good idea? What tests will be most beneficial to you and your baby? When might you want to avoid having a test done?

The information provided by these tests is less than helpful unless you understand what it means and how to use it in making decisions about your pregnancy and your medical care. Here's what the research tells us about how tests during pregnancy are done, what the results mean and when they might be helpful to you.

7

Ultrasound: Sound-Wave Images

If you have friends or relatives with babies, you've probably been treated to a showing of their ultrasound pictures. The grainy, blurred picture may not have looked much like a baby to you, even after the proud parents pointed out various body parts. Some parents have a whole series of ultrasound pictures to show off, each taken at a different stage of the pregnancy.

What is an ultrasound, and when is it useful during pregnancy?

Pregnancy ultrasound was first introduced in the 1970s, and quickly became widely available and frequently used. Improvement in ultrasound imaging equipment has been rapid—the earliest ultrasound images were not very clear, but now even subtle details of the fetus can be seen.

A pregnant woman having an ultrasound will first be asked to drink plenty of water so that her bladder is full; this isn't comfortable for the mother, but it provides the best view of the lower part of the uterus. She lies down, and warm cream is spread on her abdomen to reduce the friction of the flat, paddle-like

instrument the technician runs across her abdomen. This instrument bounces ultra high-frequency sound waves off the mother and produces an image of the fetus, placenta and uterus on a TV-like monitor beside her.

If the ultrasound is being done in early pregnancy when the uterus is still very small, a special instrument can be slipped gently into the vagina to obtain the most detailed pictures. Prints (which look like photographic negatives) can be made from the image on the monitor. These are what parents show off so proudly and paste into the front of their "baby books."

The usefulness of ultrasound to answer specific questions about a pregnancy is very clear. What is not clear is whether it is helpful for *every* pregnant woman to have an ultrasound.

Ultrasound to Answer Specific Questions

The selective ultrasound examination is done to answer a specific question. Depending on the question, the ultrasound might be done by a technician and just take a couple of minutes—such as an ultrasound done to check for twins. Another type of ultrasound might be done by a radiologist and take over an hour—such as an ultrasound done to create a biophysical profile of the baby (see Chapter 9, Tests to Assess the Baby During Pregnancy).

There are many different questions that can be answered by doing an ultrasound.

Is the Baby Alive?

Ultrasound can answer this question rapidly and accurately. If the baby's heart is beating, the baby is alive. The fetus, and its heartbeat, can be seen by seven weeks after the mother's last menstrual period.

Why is this important? If you start bleeding in the first few months of pregnancy, you can quickly find out what is going on. If the baby has died, you know that you are going to miscarry. Without an ultrasound, you might have gone through weeks of spotting and bleeding, wondering the whole time if your baby was already gone or if there was still hope that the pregnancy might continue.

Jill seemed to be having a miscarriage at about 10 weeks of pregnancy. "I was bleeding and cramping a lot and had passed some tissue. My doctor suggested doing an ultrasound just to be sure before I had a D&C [a procedure where the doctor scrapes away any remaining tissue in the uterus]. To our surprise, they found I had been pregnant with twins and only one had miscarried—the other one was doing fine. The second baby kept growing and was born at term and healthy."

How Many Weeks Pregnant Are You?

The average pregnancy lasts 40 weeks from the date of the last menstrual period. This assumes that ovulation (the release of the egg from the

What an Ultrasound Can Tell You

- Is the fetus alive (from four weeks after conception)?
- How old is the fetus (only accurate in early pregnancy)?
- Is there more than one baby?
- What is the position of the baby (is it head down, breech, etc.)?
- Are there certain abnormalities of the brain or heart (can be detected after 18 to 22 weeks)?
- How big is the baby?
- Where is the placenta?
- Is the baby growing (requires two ultrasounds at least two or three weeks apart)?

ovary) and conception occurred two weeks after menstruation began; for women with regular cycles of 28 days this assumption is usually true. For women who have very irregular periods or menstrual cycles that are longer or shorter than average, or who don't remember when their last period was, ultrasound can provide a good estimate of when their baby will be born.

The age of the baby can be estimated by ultrasound by measuring its size. In the first 12 weeks, the measurements are usually accurate to within a week. From 13 to 18 weeks of pregnancy, measurements usually predict the date of delivery to within two weeks. Measurement of the baby is not useful *at all* in predicting delivery date if it's done after 30 weeks.

Colleen had an ultrasound when she became pregnant with her second baby. Her daughter, Sophie, was 18 months old and still breastfeeding when Colleen began to suspect she had conceived again. "Because Sophie was still nursing a lot, I hadn't had a period at all since she was

Calculating Your Due Date

Your baby is considered "due" 40 weeks after the first day of your last menstrual period. To calculate this due date, take the date of your period, count back three months and add seven days.

This calculation assumes that you ovulated and conceived two weeks after the day your period started.

This calculation is quite accurate *if* you have regular 28-day menstrual cycles.

born; I really didn't think I could be pregnant," Colleen says. "But I noticed my nipples were getting sore, and I'd been feeling queasy. I did one of those drugstore tests and it came back positive. I didn't have any idea when I had gotten pregnant, so I went for an ultrasound. It told us I was 13 weeks pregnant and the baby was due around the first week of August."

Is the Baby Growing Normally?

Ultrasound is a fairly accurate way of estimating fetal size. Measurements of the head, the body and the upper leg give good estimates of the weight of the fetus at any time during the pregnancy. The individual baby's measurements can be plotted on a chart that shows the average weights at each week of pregnancy. Estimating fetal weight by ultrasound is least accurate for the biggest and the smallest babies.

However, fetal size does not show the baby's growth. A fetus who is small for gestational age through the whole pregnancy may be growing normally, even though it is smaller than average. The growth of the fetus can only be observed by doing ultrasounds two to three weeks apart.

Why might you be concerned about how fast the baby is growing? Some complications of pregnancy, such as hypertension, can cause the baby's rate of growth to slow down. If you have hypertension, your doctor may suggest having this series of ultrasounds done to see if your baby is growing normally. Another reason to check on the baby's growth might be a single ultrasound that reveals a smaller-than-average baby.

Where Is the Placenta?

The placenta looks like a large slab of liver attached along one surface to the inside of the uterus and linked by the umbilical cord to the baby. Its position gradually shifts during pregnancy and usually it ends up at the top or on one side of the uterus.

It can be a problem, though, if the placenta is across the bottom of the uterus, where the cervix is. (This is called placenta previa.) The cervix is the entrance to the vagina that the baby has to pass through to be born, and when labor contractions start to open the cervix, the placenta will be torn and will start to bleed heavily; a Caesarean section will be necessary to deliver the baby safely.

An ultrasound is the best and easiest way to determine the location of the placenta. If you have bleeding in the third trimester of pregnancy (a sign that the placenta may be at the bottom of the uterus), an ultrasound can confirm or rule out placenta previa.

This diagnosis can only be made in the third trimester of pregnancy. Many placentas are "low-lying" in early pregnancy, but move to a normal position by the end of the pregnancy.

If part of the placenta has separated from the wall of the uterus, this is called abruption of the placenta, accidental hemorrhage or premature separation of the placenta. This will cause pain and usually vaginal bleeding. An ultrasound will show where the placenta is, and the technician may be able to see blood behind the placenta or membranes. Small separations may not show up on ultrasound.

Ultrasound also makes amniocentesis and chorionic villus biopsy (tests we will discuss later) safer by showing where the placenta is, so that the biopsy needle can avoid it.

Miscellaneous Questions

There are many other specific situations in which ultrasound can be helpful during pregnancy. These include suspected twins (because of a larger-than-average uterus), suspected abnormalities in the baby (because of family history or maternal serum screening) or suspected abnormal positions of the fetus, such as breech (baby is head up instead of head down in the uterus) or transverse lie (baby is lying sideways in the uterus). Most of these will be discussed in more detail in later chapters.

Ultrasound for Everyone?

The greatest controversy surrounding ultrasound is whether it should be used on all pregnant women. Routine ultrasound will benefit pregnant women only if it shows situations that can be treated, and if this treatment will improve outcomes for mothers and babies.

Ultrasound for Everyone in the First Trimester

Ultrasound in early pregnancy is very accurate at establishing the number of weeks of pregnancy. Researchers hoped that these early pregnancy ultrasounds would reduce the number of women induced at the end of their pregnancies for being "overdue" or post-term. But the research is not conclusive—some studies found fewer inductions, others did not.

Since about 80 percent of women's expected due dates can be predicted just as accurately by their menstrual history as by

ultrasound, it is more efficient to use ultrasound selectively for women with uncertain menstrual dates.

Ultrasound for Everyone in the Third Trimester

Women who had an ultrasound in the third trimester without a specific reason showed no improvement in perinatal mortality, low Apgar score at birth or admission to the special-care nursery over women who did not have a routine ultrasound.

Benefits from routine ultrasound for everyone have not been demonstrated to date. Should we continue doing it anyway, even if there are no demonstrated benefits? There are two problems with this approach: first, while ultrasounds are apparently safe in the short term, they have not been in use long enough (or sufficiently researched) to rule out long-term harmful effects; second, every ultrasound adds to the overall cost of health care. This is reasonable and justifiable if there are benefits to mother and baby, but if no benefits can be demonstrated, the cost of routine ultrasounds is an unnecessary expense.

How Do Women Feel about Ultrasounds?

Women's feelings about ultrasounds have not been widely studied. In the studies that have been done, most women had positive feelings about having an early pregnancy ultrasound. It confirmed the reality of the baby, reduced their anxiety and increased their confidence. Some women hope to learn the sex of the child. Many like the idea of having a picture to show people. Fathers sometimes say the pregnancy feels more real to them after they see an ultrasound of the baby, and that they are reassured about the health of the baby.

**The Evidence About . . .
ULTRASOUND**

Ultrasound is very helpful to doctors and pregnant women in many specific situations.

On the other hand, the value of ultrasound for all pregnancies has not been demonstrated.

Short-term safety of ultrasound, although little researched, seems to be established. Ultrasound has not been in use long enough to identify any long-term hazards.

Parents are often not aware of the limitations of ultrasound, and assume that a "normal" ultrasound means the baby is guaranteed to be healthy (which is not the case). Not all abnormalities can be seen in a routine ultrasound.

One area that often creates anxiety is that some ultrasound technicians either are not allowed or do not wish to discuss the ultrasound results with the pregnant woman or her partner. Many women find this very frustrating and upsetting. When the person doing the ultrasound says, "I can't tell you anything, you'll have to ask your doctor," it's quite natural for the couple to react with fear and assume that something is wrong—even though the ultrasound may actually be quite normal.

Is Ultrasound Safe?

The benefit of any treatment must be weighed against the risks. There has been surprisingly little research to evaluate possible harm from ultrasound exposure to fetuses, especially considering how commonly it is used in early pregnancy. Available research is reassuring about short-term safety, although the studies have been too small to pick up any rare complications.

We do not know yet about any long-term risks, as the oldest children exposed to ultrasound are now just in their early twenties. Studies into possible long-term effects need to be done, but results will not be available for many years.

Discussing Ultrasound with Your Doctor

What if your doctor has simply assumed that you will have an ultrasound, as many do? How can you discuss this topic with him or her, if you would prefer not to have one?

- Ask if your doctor is looking for any specific information from the test. If, for example, he says he wants to confirm your due date, you can point out that you have accurate records of your last period (if you do) or other information (such as temperature charts) to determine when your baby was conceived.
- Ask your doctor what could happen if you don't have an ultrasound. What would the potential problems be? Are there other ways that these problems could be diagnosed?
- Simply tell your doctor, during an early pregnancy visit, that you would prefer not to have an ultrasound unless there is a specific reason.

8

Screening for Gestational Diabetes

Karen's first baby, Michael, weighed 10 pounds at birth. This didn't surprise her, since Karen and her husband are both tall and solidly built. Her labor with Michael was quite long, but the birth was straightforward, and he was a healthy, normal baby.

When Karen became pregnant again, her physician recommended that she be tested for gestational diabetes because her first child had been bigger than average.

"You mean I might have diabetes?" she asked.

"Gestational diabetes isn't the same as regular diabetes," her doctor explained. "It's diabetes caused by being pregnant, and it usually goes away as soon as you have the baby. But it might be a sign that you're likely to develop diabetes later in life."

Big babies can be a sign of gestational diabetes, he continued. Karen was overweight, and the doctor suggested this also might be a factor in her suspected diabetes. He warned her that babies of mothers with gestational diabetes are at risk, if the condition goes untreated.

Worried, Karen went through the glucose tolerance test her physician recommended, and the test came back "positive." She did have gestational diabetes. The doctor prescribed a strict calorie-reduced diet, which she tried hard to follow.

Two months later, the doctor met with Karen to discuss the results of the ultrasound she had had the day before to check the size of the baby.

"Have you been following the diet I gave you?"

"Most of the time," Karen said, feeling guilty about the times she had "cheated" a little and indulged in some forbidden treats.

"Well, the ultrasound shows that this is going to be another big baby."

"Bigger than Michael?"

"That depends on whether you stick to the diet. I think we should plan to induce labor about two weeks before your due date. I'll book the date at the hospital."

Karen was worried about being induced. "Is that really necessary? I've heard that induced

Laboratory Testing for Gestational Diabetes

Usually, a blood sugar test is done first when the mother has had nothing to eat (this is called a fasting blood sugar). Then the "screening" test is given—a drink containing 50 grams (1.75 oz) of sugar is taken, and the blood sugar is tested one hour later. If the result is 7.8 mm/l (0.11 fl oz/pt) or higher, the screen is considered positive. If a woman has a positive screen, a more formal test—called a glucose tolerance test—is performed. This involves drinking 100 grams (3.5 oz) of sugar and having the blood sugar tested after one, two and three hours. Upper limits of normal are 10.5 mm/l (0.15 fl oz/pt) after one hour, 9 mm/l (0.13 fl oz/pt) after two hours and 8 mm/l (0.11 fl oz/pt) after three hours. If the woman's results meet or are higher than any two of these three limits, the diagnosis of gestational diabetes is made.

labors are harder than regular ones—and won't the baby be premature?"

Her doctor waved the ultrasound report at her. "Look how big this baby is already. It'll weigh more than nine pounds even at two weeks early."

Two weeks before her due date, Karen's labor was induced. Amanda weighed 9 lbs. 8 oz. Karen found the labor difficult and used more painkillers than she had for Michael; she was also worried about her baby's health because of the diabetes. She and her husband were very relieved when the pediatrician told them Amanda was fine.

When Karen became pregnant again, the doctor recommended that she take insulin as well as follow the diet he recommended, since the diet alone clearly "hadn't worked." So

Karen took insulin injections and ate according to the doctor's instructions. She used a glucometer at home to measure her blood sugar. Even though it was usually in the normal range, she worried a lot about it. Again, the doctor's measurements and ultrasound examinations showed a larger-than-average baby, so Karen was induced two weeks before her due date. Thomas weighed 9 lb. 10 oz. and was very healthy.

Karen has three healthy children. During her first pregnancy she considered herself to be normal, but through the next two she thought of herself as "high risk" because of her gestational diabetes. Worrying about this made her last two pregnancies very stressful. She felt guilty every time she ate anything sweet or not listed on her diet sheet. She had several ultrasounds during each of her last two pregnancies to check the size of the babies. In her third pregnancy, she took insulin injections every day from 28 weeks until she was induced at 38 weeks.

What were the real risks to Karen's babies, and were these risks reduced by the treatment she received?

Gestational diabetes is glucose intolerance that appears during pregnancy. The mother feels perfectly well and healthy. The "intolerance" is not like an allergy or food intolerance that might make someone feel ill—it means that the blood sugar level is higher than average. The diagnosis is made by a laboratory, based on a "glucose tolerance test" (see sidebar) that is done between 24 and 28 weeks of pregnancy. Some doctors routinely recommend this test for all pregnant women.

About 15 percent of women who are given this test will "screen positive," and of those, about 15 percent will have a "positive" glucose tolerance test and be diagnosed with gestational diabetes. Unfortunately, this test is not very reliable. If Karen had done the test over again, it might well have come up "normal" the second time. That happens to between 50 and 70 percent of the women who are retested.

The primary risk of gestational diabetes is having a larger-than-average baby. Up to 30 percent of mothers with positive glucose tolerance tests have babies weighing more than 8 lbs. 12 oz. (4000 grams). With bigger babies, there are more Caesarean sections, and more cases where the baby's shoulders are "stuck" in the birth canal, making for a more difficult delivery.

There may be a *very small* increased risk of death of the fetus associated with an abnormal glucose tolerance test during pregnancy. However, treating women who are identified as having gestational diabetes with special diets or with insulin has *not* reduced that risk.

In Karen's case, her chance of having a bigger-than-average baby could have been predicted easily from other factors: her above-average weight before she got pregnant, the amount of weight she gained during each pregnancy, and the fact that her first baby, Michael, had been 10 pounds at birth. The glucose tolerance test didn't really tell her doctor anything he didn't already know. The test isn't even all that good at predicting who will have a larger-than-average baby: 70 percent of the mothers who test "positive" will have babies weighing less than 8 lbs. 12 oz., even with no treatment, while the majority of larger-than-average babies are born to mothers with a normal glucose test.

The low-calorie diet Karen's doctor put her on has been shown by well-designed research *not* to reduce the baby's weight at birth. Amanda was a little smaller than Michael probably just because she was a girl (and, of course, because she was delivered early). Good nutrition in pregnancy is important for all women—but good nutrition does not mean depriving yourself or being hungry.

Diabetes and Gestational Diabetes

Diabetes is a disease of high blood sugar, which develops when either the pancreas does not produce enough insulin or the cells in the body stop responding to insulin.

Type One diabetes is also called juvenile or insulin-dependent diabetes. It usually comes on fairly rapidly in young people and requires insulin treatment.

Type Two diabetes is also called adult-onset diabetes. It is strongly associated with older age, obesity and lack of physical exercise. It often comes on gradually—many people with adult-onset diabetes don't know they have it. It can sometimes be treated with a combination of nutritional changes and exercise and does not always require insulin.

Gestational diabetes or pregnancy diabetes is high blood sugar first occurring in pregnancy that goes away after the baby is born. It is associated with obesity and with developing adult-onset diabetes in later life.

Insulin treatments during pregnancy can reduce birth weight slightly, but these babies have the same risk of stillbirth, getting "stuck" shoulders or Caesarean sections as babies born to mothers diagnosed with gestational diabetes who had no treatment. Inducing labor early does not benefit either mother or baby. Caesarean sections performed solely because of the diagnosis of gestational diabetes provide no benefit to the baby and increase the risk of complications for the mother.

Since Karen had already given birth to a 10-pound baby, having another larger-than-average baby wasn't a big problem for her.

The Evidence About . . .
GESTATIONAL DIABETES

There is no benefit to either mother or baby to diagnose gestational diabetes. The diagnosis is based on an unreliable test, and the treatment with diets, insulin and early induction of labor has not been shown to help mother or baby be healthier.

There is real potential for doing more harm than good by performing a glucose tolerance test. When the test is positive, the pregnancy is likely to be considered "high risk" and the mother may undergo an expensive and extensive program of tests and treatments with no proven benefits. The anxiety produced by this diagnosis is completely out of proportion to any benefits that may be realized.

Should I Be Tested for Gestational Diabetes?

There is no benefit to routine testing for gestational diabetes for several reasons:

- The test is unreliable.
- Treatment with diet and/or insulin does not improve the outcome for the mother or the baby.
- A positive test for gestational diabetes may increase the mother's stress and anxiety levels.

What about Regular Diabetes?

It's important to understand that gestational diabetes is *not* the same as regular or overt diabetes. Overt diabetes, with high fasting blood sugar and high blood sugar after meals, is a disease that can start in childhood or adolescence and that does cause significant complications during pregnancy.

Occasionally, overt diabetes will be diagnosed for the first time during pregnancy; the symptoms are intense thirst and unusual hunger, weight loss, passing large amounts of urine and the laboratory finding of high blood sugar, both fasting and after meals. Overt diabetes requires treatment involving special diet, exercise and usually insulin therapy. This treatment would have to be continued after the baby is born as well. Pregnancy complications are higher for women with overt diabetes than for non-diabetic women; this complication rate can be improved by careful attention to blood sugar control before and during pregnancy.

Talking to Your Doctor about Gestational Diabetes

If your caregiver suggests a glucose tolerance test routinely for all her patients, and if you have decided not to be tested, you might want to bring in this section of the book for discussion. Point out that the obstetricians who wrote *Effective Care*, after carefully reviewing all the available research, do not recommend this testing.

9

Tests to Assess the Baby During Pregnancy

In This Chapter, the Following Tests Are Discussed:

1. Testing for genetic (chromosome) abnormalities
   a) chorionic villus biopsy (a sampling of the placenta done at 10–12 weeks)
   b) amniocentesis (a sampling of the amniotic fluid done at 15–18 weeks)
   c) maternal serum screening (a blood test done on the mother at 16 weeks)

2. Testing the baby's well-being
   a) ultrasound to assess size and growth
   b) biochemical tests of blood and urine
   c) fetal movement counting
   d) non-stress testing and contraction stress testing
   e) fetal biophysical profile and Doppler ultrasound

It's natural to wonder how the baby is doing while you're waiting for it to be born. (Why don't pregnant women have windows in their bellies?) Most mothers worry, at some point, whether the baby is healthy and developing normally. If someone asks you if you want a girl or a boy, you're likely to say, "I just want a healthy baby." You're probably attending your prenatal visits faithfully, primarily to be reassured that your baby is doing well.

But sometimes testing of the baby's well-being is anything but reassuring. Sharon, for example, was expecting her first baby. She was in good health and expected her pregnancy to go well. She began monthly appointments with her doctor soon after she found out she was pregnant, and was put through a set of testing and assessment procedures that her doctor assured her was "routine." First, the doctor suggested an ultrasound to "confirm her dates," even though Sharon keeps careful track of her menstrual cycles and knew when her last period was. Then she had the maternal serum screening, which placed her in the "high-risk" group, followed by an amniocentesis to see if her baby had Down syndrome (it didn't). By the time Sharon actually went into labor, she'd had three more ultrasounds to make sure her baby was growing normally, and had been through a "stress test" to see if her baby would be able to cope with labor.

Sharon's experience may not be typical, but it's certainly not uncommon. And now Sharon definitely feels anxious about pregnancy and birth. She's spent a lot of time worrying about this baby and sees it as a vulnerable little person in a risky situation. Sharon's extra stress (and the costs of her tests to the medical system) will be worth it if the procedures help her to have a healthier baby. Will they? That's the question researchers have tried to answer as they've looked at various methods of assessing the baby before birth.

How can parents and professionals determine if the baby is, in fact, growing as it should be and doing well? In the past, mothers watched their abdomens grow larger each month and felt the baby move. That didn't provide a lot of information, but it did show that the baby was alive and getting bigger. Since the late 1960s, several methods of assessing the health of the fetus have been developed. These tests can be used for women with health problems that make their babies more at risk of certain problems, or they can be offered to all pregnant women.

Testing for Genetic Abnormalities

Some of the tests diagnose chromosomal (genetic) abnormalities in the fetus. There are no treatments for these problems, but you can consider a therapeutic abortion if the fetus is found to be abnormal.

Abortion is a topic that generates strong emotions, and the decision about whether to have an abortion is a very personal one. Some parents choose to have these tests done because they know that if the fetus is abnormal, they will have an abortion. Parents who would not choose an abortion may still want to know if their child has genetic abnormalities, to help them to prepare. In any case, parents who choose to have any of these screening tests done should spend some time beforehand discussing what they will do if their baby does have a genetic abnormality. How do they feel about abortion? How do they feel about caring for a disabled child?

Chorionic Villus Biopsy and Amniocentesis

Chorionic villus biopsy is a method of obtaining fetal cells early in pregnancy (10 to 12 weeks) to test for any chromosome abnormality (such as Down syndrome). To perform this test, a needle is inserted either through the mother's abdomen into the uterus, or more often through the vagina and cervix into the uterus, to take a sample from the chorion (cells developing into the placenta). Ultrasound is used to help the doctor guide the needle to the right place. Since these cells are actually part of the baby, they can be examined to see if there are any chromosome abnormalities.

Chorionic villus biopsy is done before 12 weeks of pregnancy. This is an advantage for women who may decide to have an abortion if there is a chromosome abnormality, because abortion is a simpler procedure at this point. However, many fetuses with chromosomal abnormalities spontaneously miscarry early in the pregnancy. If the mother had opted to wait and have amniocentesis instead, she might have miscarried the baby before the time for the testing arrived.

Amniocentesis is the withdrawal of a small amount of amniotic fluid from the uterus by a needle (again, with ultrasound images to help the doctor get the needle in exactly the right place). This fluid contains cells from the fetus, and these are analyzed for chromosomal defects (such as Down syndrome and other, more rare chromosome abnormalities). Amniocentesis is done between 15 and 18 weeks of pregnancy and the analysis takes two or three weeks. This can be significant if an abnormality is found and the mother decides to have an abortion, as the pregnancy will now be between 17 and 19 weeks. This makes the abortion itself more complicated, and it can be more emotionally distressing for the mother than if it was done during the first trimester.

Mothers over the age of 35 are most likely to have this test done because they are, statistically, at higher-than-average risk of having a child with a chromosome abnormality. You may also be offered the test if you have already had a child with a chromosome abnormality, or if you have a close relative with an abnormality.

Amniocentesis will also be offered to women who get a "positive" result on the maternal serum screening for Down syndrome, but it will not be offered to those who screen negative (see next section).

What are the risks of these procedures? Chorionic villus biopsies and amniocentesis both have a low complication rate. Chorionic villus biopsy needs a repeat test (because the first one didn't give clear results) in a little more than 2 percent of cases. Amniocentesis needs to be repeated between 1 and 2 percent of the time. The actual rate of failure varies with the experience of the center doing the testing. The rate of miscarriage after amniocentesis is about 1 in 200, and the risk of a very low birth weight baby or a baby with breathing problems is also about 1 in 200. Chorionic villus biopsy has a higher rate of pregnancy loss than amniocentesis, but the exact risk is very difficult to state because many studies include abortions as well as miscarriages in the pregnancy loss numbers. For both procedures,

Testing for Gene Abnormalities

Chromosome testing looks for abnormalities in the 46 chromosomes (23 pairs) in our cells. The most common of these is Down syndrome, in which the affected person has three of chromosome 21, instead of two.

Genes are the thousands of tiny subunits on each chromosome that control our bodies in many different ways. We now know that many diseases (like sickle cell anemia, hemophilia, muscular dystrophy, cystic fibrosis and others) are controlled by a single identifiable faulty gene. These genes are *not* tested for in routine amniocentesis or chorionic villus biopsy, but if requested because of a specific family history of the disease, these genes can be identified by these tests.

complication rates seem to be lowest at testing centers with the most experience.

Regardless of your situation, you can simply decline these tests if you prefer not to have them done. Some women know they don't want to have an abortion even if the baby has Down syndrome or other problems. They feel that having a positive test result will make the pregnancy more stressful and are more comfortable just waiting to see what happens.

Maternal Serum Screening
"When you come back next month you will be 16 weeks along, and we can do the maternal serum screening," says your doctor.

"What's that?"

"Just a blood test. It will tell us if the baby is okay."

You are handed a pamphlet to read as you walk out wondering what this test is all about.

Informed Consent

Informed consent is an important part of ethical medical care, but it can be harder to achieve than it sounds. If a medical test (or a medical treatment) is offered or recommended, you should be given information about the test that allows you to decide whether you want to have it done.

That sounds straightforward. But when you are pregnant, you generally have to rely on your doctor or midwife as the source of information, and it's easy for them to present even accurate information in a slanted or biased manner. They may emphasize the risks or the potential benefits, for example.

In some cases—and maternal serum screening is one of them—the information is fairly complicated and can take a long time to explain.

To be truly informed about prenatal tests and other aspects of your medical care, you may want to seek additional sources of information such as books like this one, your childbirth educator, Internet resources or a genetic counselor.

Most of the pregnant women you know have had it done, and the doctor certainly seems to think it's just routine. It might be reassuring to know that the baby is healthy....

Maternal serum screening (MSS) does not "tell you if the baby is okay." It is a screening test, which means that it tells you the chance of your baby having certain abnormalities. It does *not* tell you whether your baby, in fact, does have these abnormalities.

MSS is a popular test, primarily because it is simple to do; it is almost routinely offered to all pregnant women in Ontario, for example. It isn't, however, simple to explain, and when the information is simplified it is usually not accurate and leaves out important details. Before deciding to have this test done, you should understand the information the test can provide.

To perform the MSS test, a sample of the mother's blood is taken when she is between 15 and 17 weeks pregnant. It is very important for the accuracy of the results that the dates be precise. This sample is then analyzed in a lab. There is no risk to either mother or baby when the test is done.

The test determines the probability of two separate abnormalities in your baby. One is Down syndrome, a chromosome abnormality that causes mental retardation and can cause physical problems in the baby as well (MSS also screens for trisomy 18—a much more rare chromosome abnormality). The other is an abnormality in the development of the baby's brain or spinal cord called an open neural tube defect. This can be either anencephaly, in which the baby's brain does not develop (and the baby will not live), or spina bifida, in which the spinal cord does not fuse. Spina bifida can cause different degrees of disability, from complete paralysis below the waist to varying degrees of leg weakness.

The test does *not* tell you whether your baby has one of these problems. Instead, it tells you the relative chance of your baby having either Down syndrome or a neural tube defect. The results for the two tests are determined from the same blood sample, but are quite separate. If your results fall into a risk category above a certain level for either abnormality, this is called a "high-risk" or "positive" screen.

In the general population, the overall risk of any woman having a baby with a neural tube defect is 1 or 2 per 1000 pregnancies. For women who have already had a baby with a neural tube defect, or who have a close family relative with this condition, the risk increases to 10 per 1000. Calculating the risk of Down syndrome is more complicated because it increases with the mother's age: at age 20, the risk of having a baby with Down syndrome is 1 in 1200; at age 40, the risk is 1 in 100. Also, a woman who has already had a baby with Down syndrome has a higher risk of having another baby with Down syndrome.

The MSS test results come back to your doctor as a number (1 out of 1000, for example, or 1 out of 210), which is your chance of having a baby with that abnormality. In Ontario, the "positive" or "high-risk" screen for Down syndrome has been defined arbitrarily as a risk of 1 in 385 or greater. So, a risk of 1 in 400 would be negative, while a risk of 1 in 300 would be positive. A "positive" or "high-risk" screen for neural tube defects has been defined arbitrarily as a risk of 1 in 100. Women who screen positive for these abnormalities are offered further testing.

Obviously, a "positive" screen does not mean that your baby has the problem being tested for—as the numbers show, in almost all cases the baby does not. On the other hand, a "negative" screen does not mean that the baby *won't* have these problems—the MSS will screen "positive" for only 70 percent of Down syndrome cases and 80 percent of open neural tube defects.

Deciding what the results of the test mean for you as an individual can be very difficult. What can you do to clarify the situation if your test is "positive," as it is for about 8 percent of those tested?

You can, if you like, have further testing to follow up on these results. First, you should confirm the exact accuracy of your dates. If you were less than 16 weeks pregnant when the test was done, you could repeat the test at between 16 and 18 weeks. This might give you more accurate results.

If your screen is "positive" for Down syndrome, you can have an amniocentesis, which

can give you a definite answer about whether your baby has this condition, but which also carries a risk of miscarriage of about 1 in 200. Detailed ultrasound is increasingly used to detect physical signs of Down syndrome in the fetus.

If your test is "positive" for neural tube defect, you can have a detailed ultrasound, which will diagnose anencephaly and possibly spina bifida. You can also have the serum AFP repeated or have an amniocentesis to test the AFP (Alpha-Fetoprotein) levels in the amniotic fluid—if these tests are positive, the risk of a neural tube defect is higher.

Parents should also recognize that no test guarantees a perfect baby. Tracy says, "I had the MSS test done, and was so reassured when the results came back low risk. I thought they meant the baby was healthy. It shocked me when he was born and had a rare condition that causes developmental delays and other physical handicaps. His syndrome doesn't show up on the test." Remember as well that 30 percent of babies with Down syndrome are born to mothers whose MSS tests came back negative.

Katherine had the MSS done for the first time when she was pregnant with her fourth child. She decided to have the screening because she was now 36, and her doctor advised her that she had a higher risk of having a baby with Down syndrome. When the test came back "positive," Katherine and her husband didn't know what to do. "Did it mean we had a baby with Down syndrome? I asked the doctor. No, just that I was in a higher-risk group. Well, I knew I was in a higher-risk group because of my age, so that wasn't very helpful. We couldn't figure out what this meant. I was confused, Jack was confused, we didn't know what we should do next."

After discussing it with her husband and her doctor, Katherine decided to repeat the test. Again, the results were "positive." The doctor explained Katherine's options, but none of them appealed to her very much. Even if she had an amniocentesis and found out that the baby had Down syndrome, she wasn't sure that having an abortion would be a possible choice for her. "It already felt like a real baby to me," she says.

Katherine decided not to have an amniocentesis, but she continued to worry about her baby. To her relief, Devon was born quite normal and healthy. "We hadn't really thought it out enough," she says now. "We had the test because the doctor recommended it, but Jack and I never discussed what we'd do if the test came back 'positive.'"

What does it mean if your test is "negative"? It doesn't mean that your baby is guaranteed to be normal. This test only covers two possible conditions, and your baby might have some other problem. It is also possible that your baby will have either Down syndrome or an open neural tube defect, even though your test was "negative." The "negative" test simply means that you have a lower chance of a baby with these problems.

What does it mean if your baby does have one of the disabilities mentioned? Both Down syndrome and open neural tube defects have a range of severities. Some people with Down syndrome, for example, have serious disabilities; others lead productive and happy lives with some assistance. The tests can't tell you how severe—or how mild—the problem will be.

Even if you initially requested the screening because you planned to have an abortion if the results were "positive," you can change your mind. You also may decide that an abortion is the right choice for you and your family even though it hadn't seemed like an option before you had any tests done. Counseling to discuss your options is available; you also might want to contact one of the support groups for parents of children with Down syndrome or neural tube problems to get a realistic picture of the range of disability.

Just because a test is easy to do doesn't mean it should be done. Before you choose to have maternal serum screening, be sure you understand what it is testing for and the uncertainty of the results. Discuss with your partner beforehand whether you will have further testing if you have a positive screen result. It's also important to discuss your feelings about abortion, even if you don't make a hard and fast decision, because if abortion is being considered, further testing must occur immediately.

How Is the Baby Doing in the Uterus?

Beyond these tests for genetic problems, which can be diagnosed but can't be treated, physicians and researchers have looked for ways to assess the baby's health as it grows inside the uterus. The goal is a two-part one: to find ways of determining which babies are not growing well before birth, and to find effective ways of improving the situation for those babies.

Measuring the Size and Growth of the Fetus

One of the things that doctors and researchers try to determine is the size of the baby. Their concerns are that a very big baby might be prone to problems if it doesn't fit through the mother's pelvis at birth; a very small baby may be weak, malnourished and not able to cope with the stress of labor and birth. This isn't always true: some women give birth without difficulty to large babies, and some babies are just meant to be smaller than average.

At each prenatal visit, you will probably have your abdomen measured from your pubic bone to the top of the uterus. This is called the fundal height. Is this an accurate measurement? If you have two doctors measure your abdomen, they're likely to come up with different numbers. However, despite these limitations, the method does predict fairly accurately which babies will be large and which will be very small.

Ultrasound is much more reliable in measuring the size of the baby. Researchers have done hundreds of ultrasounds at various stages of pregnancy, measured the fetuses and worked out the expected average size of the baby for every week of pregnancy. These charts of average weights have become the "gold standard" for assessing situations where the fetus is thought to be too small.

If your baby seems to be smaller than expected when your abdomen is measured, your caregiver will probably recommend an ultrasound to check the baby's size more accurately.

However, there is a big difference between fetal *size* and fetal *growth*. Assessing the size of the fetus can be done with one ultrasound. The technician looks at the baby, measures it and compares it to the average. To determine how the baby is growing requires at least two ultrasounds performed long enough apart for the baby to have grown.

When the fetus is below the 10th percentile of the average weights determined by ultrasound, it is described as "light for dates," "small for dates" or "small for gestational age." If you are told that your baby is "small for dates," you will probably feel very concerned. Is your baby in trouble? Not necessarily. Not all small babies are small for the same reasons.

For example, your baby may simply be meant to be small. Perhaps you weighed less than six pounds at birth, even though you were full-term, and your brother was two ounces smaller than you when he arrived. In this case, it's not surprising that the baby you are carrying is also a bit smaller than average, and it will likely remain small throughout your pregnancy.

Some babies are smaller than average because they have picked up an infection such as rubella or toxoplasmosis early in the pregnancy. This is a concern, but there is no treatment that will make these babies bigger or healthier.

Another group of babies start out growing at an average rate, but then their rate of growth begins to lag behind. A baby in this group is not necessarily "small for dates." For example, if the fetus was at the 90th percentile and has now dropped to the 40th percentile, it would still be considered within the normal, average range of size. However, the dramatic drop in growth means the fetus is probably at some risk—there is likely a problem that has caused this sudden change. It is impossible to tell if your baby is in this group unless you have at least two ultrasounds. If your baby's growth has slowed down, it is described as having "intra-uterine growth restriction." Most researchers believe this is caused by a problem with the blood supply to the placenta, which is preventing the baby from getting enough nutrition. This situation can be dangerous for your baby, who is at a higher risk of serious problems before, during and after birth. The baby's risk of health problems during childhood and adult life is also higher.

What can be done to help these babies?

- Smoking: Many babies with intra-uterine growth restriction have mothers who smoke. If you quit smoking, your baby's rate of growth will improve.
- Nutrition: If you are thin and undernourished, you have a higher risk of having a low birth weight baby. However, eating more will only cause a slight improvement in your baby's growth. This probably means that women need to be eating well before they conceive to help their babies grow.
- Bed rest: Women with small babies have been advised to rest in bed, but there is no evidence that bed rest helps the baby to grow.
- Abdominal decompression: One interesting approach uses abdominal decompression as

a way of increasing the blood flow to the placenta. A large plastic dome is placed over the woman's abdomen and the air is pumped out, leaving a partial vacuum over her abdomen. If this technique is used repeatedly during pregnancy with a small for dates baby, studies show a significant increase in birth weight (on average, more than a pound). This method has not found its way into mainstream medicine because it was introduced with unfounded claims of benefit for all babies, not just small ones. Larger studies would provide a better evaluation of this approach, which seems to have potential. If your baby has intra-uterine growth restriction, you could certainly ask your doctor if this option is available where you live.

- Drugs: Another potentially helpful treatment is the use of calcium channel blockers and betamimetics. Some small studies have shown promising results, but larger studies need to be done before these medications can be recommended.
- Induction of labor: It is common for doctors to suggest induction of labor as soon as the pregnancy is far enough along that prematurity is not a major risk. The theory is that the baby will grow better on the outside than it currently is on the inside. The timing of induction has not been studied enough to make any recommendations and additional research is needed. At present, each situation must be evaluated individually.

Biochemical Tests

Tests of various enzymes and hormones in the mother's blood and urine have been done at different times since the 1960s to predict fetuses who were in distress. This testing was usually done on mothers with complications: diabetes, high blood pressure or pregnancies that had gone well past the due date. If the levels varied from normal, labor was often induced.

Unfortunately, when babies born to mothers who had been given these tests were compared with babies whose mothers had not been tested, there was no difference in outcomes.

Fetal Movement Counting

The baby who is not doing well in the uterus may move much less for a day or so before it dies. Knowing this, some researchers suggested that pregnant women count how often the baby kicked for a set time period each day. If the baby wasn't moving as much as it had in the past, the mother would call her doctor, and tests would be done to find out what was going on with the baby.

This was such a simple, easily done test that it became very popular. However, when the research studies were completed, they found that counting the baby's movements did not improve the outcomes. Even worse, when the mother reported that her baby was moving less frequently, she was likely to undergo further testing, be admitted to hospital and have labor induced. Each of these procedures has complications and costs, and there were no overall benefits to the babies.

Non-stress Testing

In the 1960s, electronic fetal monitors (EFM) were introduced into the care of pregnant women. The EFM measures the baby's heartbeat through the mother's abdomen and records it on a continuous printout.

While the EFM is most often used in labor, a "non-stress" test for pregnant women was soon developed. The EFM belts are strapped across the woman's belly, and the machine records the baby's heartbeat for 20 minutes.

What are the doctors looking for? A normal or "reactive" test shows the baby's heartbeat occasionally speeding up and slowing down, rather than staying the same all the time. If the baby kicks, or if the mother drinks something cold, you would expect to see an acceleration in the heart rate.

Researchers hoped that a "reactive" test would show that the baby was healthy and likely to do well through the rest of pregnancy and during labor. (If the baby's non-stress tests were not reactive, the doctor might intervene, most often by inducing labor.) However, the number of babies who died was actually higher in the study groups where doctors had access to the non-stress test results than in the control groups where doctors did not have this information.

Diana says, "I think the name 'non-stress' test is inaccurate. It was pretty stressful for me! Having to go down to the hospital, wait until I was called, lie there while they ran the monitor and then wait while they studied the results was not my idea of a good way to spend an afternoon. I worried the whole time the monitor was running. Some days they would leave it running for a long time and I would think that something was wrong, and then my nurse would tell me she got held up with another patient. Then she would say, 'It looks fine today—but your doctor wants you to come back and have another one next week'—so I never really stopped worrying. It's discouraging to realize that, after all I went through, my doctor really didn't get any useful information."

Contraction Stress Testing

The contraction stress test is also called an "oxytocin challenge test." It is done exactly the same way as a non-stress test, except that the mother is given the drug oxytocin (through an IV) to cause contractions.

Just as in the non-stress test, the doctor is looking to see if the baby's heartbeat changes when there is a contraction. This test is performed at or near the end of pregnancy, and is intended to determine which babies will cope well with labor and which will be at risk of problems or death during labor.

However, studies showed that there were no benefits for the babies. Any information the test gave did not help the doctors in delivering the babies safely.

Fetal Biophysical Profile

The biophysical profile of the fetus is a specialized ultrasound that looks at five things: fetal movement, muscle tone, breathing movements, heart rate and the volume of amniotic fluid. It provides more information than just recording the baby's heartbeat does.

The test is more useful in one way: it does a better job than the previous tests of predicting which babies will get into trouble during labor. Unfortunately, using the profile did not result in better outcomes for the babies in the small studies done so far. This is a good area to research further, as at least the test does identify babies at risk.

Doppler Ultrasound

This method of checking on the baby *can* be helpful in some specific cases. The Doppler ultrasound can be used to measure the amount of blood flowing through the umbilical artery (the major blood vessel in the umbilical cord, carrying nutrients and oxygen from the placenta to the baby).

Doing this test routinely on all pregnancies did not lead to better outcomes for the babies. However, when the test was done on mothers who had high blood pressure and babies who had intra-uterine growth restriction, it was very good at picking out which babies were seriously at risk of problems during labor and birth. (These babies are at a higher risk anyway, because of the hypertension or growth restriction, but the Doppler ultrasound narrows it down still further.) Delivering the babies at risk right away has been shown to reduce the number of babies who die or suffer other complications.

The Evidence About...
ASSESSING THE BABY DURING PREGNANCY

The more sophisticated ultrasound techniques do identify fetuses at risk, so there is hope that treatments to improve the outcomes for these babies will be found.

Selectively using Doppler ultrasound on certain women has been demonstrated to improve outcomes for these babies.

---

tion has been demonstrated to improve the outcomes for mothers and babies.

We've also learned that:

- Recognizing situations where the fetus is at risk does not always mean there is anything we can do to reduce that risk.
- Large-scale clinical trials to assess the effectiveness of these tests and interventions should be done *first*, before they become widely used on pregnant women.

Discussing Tests During Pregnancy with Your Doctor

Some tests—for example, the MSS—are offered routinely by many doctors. Others will be recommended if you fit certain categories. For example, your doctor may recommend an amniocentesis if you are over 35, or a biophysical profile if you have gone more than a week past your due date.

You can weigh your doctor's recommendation against the research results cited in this book, and decide whether you want to have the test.

You may want to have an amniocentesis even though you have ruled out the option of abortion, for example, because you would like time to prepare for a disabled child. Or you may have decided that you would rather not know, and can therefore tell your doctor that you don't want any of these screening tests.

What if your doctor wants to have a biophysical profile done? You can ask how the information obtained will be used, and let him know that you are concerned that research hasn't shown any benefits to this procedure—other than predicting which babies are more likely to have problems.

Prenatal Fetal Assessment: What Have We Learned?

If you're feeling a little discouraged as you read this section, you're not alone. The research summarized here is pretty disappointing.

Everyone involved in caring for pregnant women—and, of course, the expectant parents themselves—would like to be able to identify potential problems and solve them so that more babies are born healthy. A number of methods of testing the well-being of the fetus have been introduced, and some have been used very widely. Many have been used as the basis for making decisions about care for the pregnant woman and her baby. Yet a careful assessment of the research and clinical trials shows that most of these tests have not improved the outcome for babies.

In many cases, we got more information. We learned a lot about the fetus and placenta from the biochemical tests. We learned a lot about fetal growth and development from ultrasound. But, so far, little of this informa-

10

"High-Risk Pregnancy"

Is your pregnancy low or high risk?

Before considering the factors that may lead you to be classified as one or the other, it's important to look at what "high risk" means.

Jennifer says, "I thought being 'high risk' meant the baby had a high probability of developing problems. And to me that means definitely more than a 50 percent chance, maybe more than an 80 percent chance. I was shocked when I discovered that being high risk for beta strep infection, for example, means about a 2 percent chance of the baby having it. Or that being high risk for Down syndrome is still less than 1 percent."

Because of this very common misunderstanding about what "high risk" means, it is often better to think of "higher-than-average risk" or some other less worrying phrase.

The decision about your risk level matters because it will affect the kind of care you receive and the options you have. If you are low risk, you may be able to give birth at home or in a birthing center, with a midwife or a family physician. If you are considered to be high risk, you may be referred to an obstetrician and advised to go to a larger hospital for your baby's birth.

But knowing your relative risk level is only helpful if it means you and your baby are likely to do better as a result. Current methods of determining which mothers are "at risk"—usually just scoring the answers to a list of questions based on the mother's past medical history—are not very helpful.

Depending on the criteria used, somewhere between 10 and 30 percent of the mothers labeled high risk will actually experience any of the problems the risk screening process is supposed to highlight. A significant number (between 20 and 50 percent, again depending on the criteria used) of the babies who have problems (specifically prematurity or low birth weight) will be born to mothers who were rated low risk. In other words, the factors used to divide women into low- or high-risk groups are not very reliable.

Judith and her husband had not been able to conceive after two years of trying, so they saw a fertility specialist who diagnosed the problem as a low sperm count and irregular ovulation. After several months of treatments, Judith still wasn't pregnant, so they decided to "take a break" from trying to conceive. To their delight, Judith discovered she was pregnant three months later.

"I called the fertility specialist to let him know we were pregnant and wouldn't be coming back, and said I was planning to return to my family doctor for my prenatal care and the birth of the baby. The doctor called me back and said that because I had fertility problems I was high risk and needed to be cared for by an obstetrician," says Judith.

Judith and her husband discussed the situation, and decided to return to their family doctor. As Judith says, "We'd had trouble conceiving, but I couldn't see why this made me a high risk. And in the end, we'd gotten pregnant on our own, without the treatments. This was just a normal pregnancy." Judith eventually gave birth to a nine-pound baby boy in the birthing center connected to her hospital.

Even if you have been accurately described as "high risk"—meaning you and your baby *are* at a higher risk for certain problems—knowing this is not very helpful if nothing can be done about it. Many of the factors can't be changed, and there are not always interventions that can improve the outcome.

In fact, in many studies, being labeled "high risk" meant that mothers were subjected to a number of additional interventions, and often these were not helpful. Since all interventions carry some risk, it would make more sense to minimize interventions as much as possible for high-risk pregnancies.

Being told you are "high risk" also means added stress for you and your family.

Often women are classified as "high risk" simply because they are part of a group. If you are a teenager, or a woman over 40, you might be told that you are "high risk" because of your age, even though this classification has little to do with you as an individual. Or you might be described as "high risk" because of the number of children you have, as Cally discovered.

When Cally became pregnant with her seventh child, her family doctor, who had delivered her previous six babies, told her she was now "high risk" and should see an obstetrician. This didn't make sense to Cally. "I had no problems at all with the previous six pregnancies and births," she said. "I keep fit, I'm healthy, and I couldn't see any reason why the last pregnancy would be low risk and suddenly this one was high risk." She persuaded her family doctor to continue providing her prenatal care and to attend the birth, which was as straightforward as her previous ones had been.

There are also plenty of gray areas, where women are not actually at any higher risk of problems but may be close enough to whatever definition of "high risk" is being used to cause comment. When Keshia was pregnant, her doctor was concerned that Keshia's blood pressure was "borderline." At each prenatal appointment, the doctor discussed the interventions that would be suggested if her blood pressure went any higher. Keshia found this very stressful, especially when her doctor talked about inducing labor. Finally, she asked the doctor to put the discussion of possible treatments "on hold" until her blood pressure actually changed. It never did.

What if you do fall into the category of higher-than-average risk (remember, that could mean you have a 1 or 2 percent chance of certain problems)? You may be in this category because you have a medical problem, such as diabetes that is not well controlled, or because you have high blood pressure. You may have a complicated pregnancy—perhaps you are expecting triplets, or the baby is growing more slowly than expected. You may simply be older than the average mother, which places you at greater risk of having a baby with Down syndrome or having a Caesarean section.

The high-risk label is not very helpful unless it improves the outcome for you and your baby. As a "high-risk" mother, what do you need?

1. Information about what aspects of your pregnancy are "high risk" and what (if anything) can be done to lower the risk, including minimizing interventions.
2. Information about how you can prepare for possible complications (for example, a premature baby).

3. Extra emotional support during pregnancy and birth.

Often, women who are considered to be high risk find that in labor they are surrounded by medical personnel—most of them strangers—rather than their partners, friends and others who can provide comfort and emotional support. While there may be a need for extra technology, this doesn't diminish the need for emotional support. It may be helpful to hire a doula to be with you at this time, or to make arrangements with your hospital and doctor to bring extra support people with you.

Who Is at Higher Risk?

Early on in your pregnancy, you may be asked questions such as these to determine your risk level:

* How old are you? (oldest and youngest ages are higher risk)
* How much do you weigh? (obese women are at a higher risk)
* Do you have any medical problems, such as diabetes, epilepsy, high blood pressure, HIV positive status, heart disease, blood clotting disorders, etc.?
* Have you had any complications during your previous pregnancies? (some of these may recur, such as high blood pressure, postpartum hemorrhage, premature birth)

During your pregnancy, things may happen that place you in the higher-than-average risk group:

* vaginal bleeding;
* developing high blood pressure;
* premature leaking of the amniotic fluid;
* premature labor;
* smaller- or larger-than-usual weight gain or fetal size;
* being diagnosed with an infection;
* carrying more than one baby.

Remember: *Identifying risk factors does not necessarily mean that anything can be done about them.*

Part Three

Pregnancy Problems

Adrienne Leong

After all you'd heard about pregnant women glowing, you're finding you mostly look green. Why do they call it "morning sickness" when it seems to last all day? And you hate waking up in the middle of the night with terrible cramps in your leg. Your complaints seem minor, though, when you talk to your friend who has already suffered through a couple of bladder infections and now has high blood pressure.

There are both common discomforts during pregnancy and more unusual symptoms that might require extra medical care. You might also be concerned about the position your baby is lying in while inside your uterus, or about being Rh negative.

Here's the best evidence about some of the common—and not-so-common—problems you may experience during pregnancy.

The Discomforts of Pregnancy

Pregnancy is a state of health, not disease. Yet pregnancy often brings with it symptoms that at any other time might be considered signs of illness. Elizabeth, a physician, remembers that when she was three months pregnant, "I was sure I had a brain tumor. I knew I was pregnant as well, but I didn't believe that just being pregnant could cause such bad headaches, or make me vomit so much. I kept thinking—my poor baby, after I die of my brain tumor, it will have no mother. Not very rational, I now realize, but that was how awful I felt."

Few studies have looked at treatments for the so-called "minor" symptoms of pregnancy. Yet some symptoms are fairly common, and may make women feel too unwell to go to work, or to take care of their homes and families.

Because pregnancy symptoms obviously go away either during or after pregnancy, almost any treatment is going to appear to "work" some of the time. To really see if a treatment is effective, we need controlled studies in which the treatment is measured against either another treatment or doing nothing at all.

Discomforts versus Dangers

Many uncomfortable and unpleasant symptoms during pregnancy are normal and don't indicate any serious problems. However, some signs should be promptly checked out with your caregiver:

- Vaginal bleeding, especially in the last few months of pregnancy
- Severe or persistent headache, especially in late pregnancy
- Flashing lights or spots before your eyes, especially in late pregnancy
- Sudden increase in swelling of hands, face or feet
- Leaking of amniotic fluid
- Not feeling the baby move for 24 hours
- Severe or persistent abdominal pain
- Significant fever

Morning Sickness

Watch any soap opera; if one of the characters rushes into the bathroom to throw up, or complains of a queasy feeling at breakfast, you know the pregnancy test is going to be positive. "Morning sickness" is so common and such a well-known symptom that pregnant women who don't feel nauseated are surprised.

"Morning sickness" isn't the best name for it. While some women are especially queasy when they first wake up in the morning, others feel sick all day long. At least half of pregnant women experience some nausea, with or without actual vomiting, in early pregnancy. (Feeling queasy is much more common than actually vomiting.) For a small percentage of women, vomiting is so severe that they become dehydrated and lose weight. This is called hyperemesis (which means excessive vomiting). These women may need to be hospitalized temporarily to be given intravenous fluids.

Elizabeth says, "This is how it went every morning for about two months: I'd get out of bed, rush to the bathroom and throw up. Then I'd have a shower, and get out just in time to throw up again. I'd get dressed, stagger downstairs and try to eat a little toast, even though I was feeling terrible. Usually I'd throw the toast up as soon as I got to the office. But by lunch-time it was usually a bit better, and I could eat a little more. Then I could usually eat a normal supper."

The cause or causes of nausea and vomiting during pregnancy are not yet known. This has hindered the development of effective treatments. For women who have mild nausea and queasiness, eating small, frequent meals may be the best way to reduce unpleasant feelings. (This can be easier said than done for women who have to go to work and may not have easy access to quick snacks.) Other treatments that have been studied are discussed below.

Acupressure

Two small studies looked at acupressure on a specific point (P6) on the mother's wrist. While the studies were small, they both found that the acupressure significantly reduced nausea. Since this treatment doesn't involve any drugs and harmful effects are unlikely, it's something pregnant women could consider trying. Wrist straps sold for carsickness and seasickness are widely available in drugstores and will put pressure on the appropriate area of the mother's wrist.

Dietary Supplements

Ginger has been shown to reduce nausea, and one small study found that extra vitamin B_6 was also helpful. Mothers can easily add these to their diet, either by changing what they eat or taking supplements.

Medications for Nausea

A number of medications to stop severe vomiting in early pregnancy have been tested.

Bendectin was once the most widely prescribed drug in pregnancy, and studies showed it was highly effective in treating nausea and vomiting. The manufacturers took it off the market in 1983 because of lawsuits by parents whose babies were born with abnormalities after the mothers had taken Bendectin. Since a certain percentage of birth defects always occurs in the general population, and because Bendectin was so frequently prescribed, it was inevitable that some babies whose mothers had taken the drug would be born with birth defects. That doesn't mean that Bendectin *caused* the problem, and, in fact, 19 large studies showed that mothers who took Bendectin had no higher risk of babies with birth defects than mothers who didn't take it. However, the drug company did not want to fight all the lawsuits and decided to stop selling Bendectin. It is unfortunate that this effective and safe medication became unavailable to pregnant women.

Diclectin combines doxylamine (an antihistamine) and pyridoxine (vitamin B_6). It is the only drug licensed by the Health Protection Branch (Canada) to be sold specifically to treat nausea and vomiting during pregnancy. Interestingly, its ingredients are two of the three drugs that were in Bendectin.

Antihistamines are commonly used to treat nausea and vomiting. They are effective, and although their safety has not been as widely studied as was done for Bendectin, there is no evidence that they cause any harm.

Heartburn

Heartburn is a common problem for pregnant women. It can be reduced to a certain extent by avoiding high-fat or spicy foods and by not lying down immediately after eating. If those measures don't help enough, any of the antacids available in drugstores can be tried, as research has found they cause no harm to the baby. Lemon juice or acidic lemonade can also be tried.

Elevating the head of the bed to sleep can also reduce heartburn. This does not mean sleeping on more pillows, which can actually make heartburn worse. Instead, put blocks under the head of the bed (or insert a wedge between the mattress and the box spring) to put the whole bed on a slight slant.

Constipation

Women who tend to be constipated when not pregnant usually experience worse constipation with pregnancy.

Eating lots of fruit, vegetables, beans, whole grains and bran, drinking more water and get-

ting more exercise helps constipation in one-third of pregnant women.

If constipation persists after trying these remedies, laxatives can be used. The safest laxatives to use during pregnancy are the ones that are either "bulking agents" or "stool softeners" (ask your caregiver to recommend a brand name). These are not absorbed into the body, will not affect the baby and can be used safely throughout pregnancy. Other laxatives irritate the bowel, are absorbed into the body and cross the placenta. These should be used only on a short-term basis, if at all, because their safety in pregnancy has not been established.

Iron supplements can cause constipation. Since iron supplements have not been shown to be helpful during pregnancy (see Chapter 5, Nutrition and Exercise), if you are taking iron and suffering from constipation, stopping the supplements may help.

Fatigue

Many women feel extremely tired, particularly during the early months of pregnancy, even if they are not anemic or malnourished. Minimal research has been done on this symptom. Apparently, creating a baby uses a lot of energy and the only treatment is rest and time.

Yeast Infection

Yeast infections of the vagina are common in non-pregnant women, and are two to ten times more common during pregnancy. Yeast vaginitis can cause a heavy, white, curdy discharge, itching and a sore, tender vagina, but it will not infect the uterus, harm the baby or cause any pregnancy complications.

If yeast is causing soreness or itching, it is safe to treat it with vaginal suppositories or cream containing either imidazole or nystatin. Imidazole has been found to be more effective than nystatin. There is a tendency for yeast to come back again, even after treatment, and the treatment can be repeated during the pregnancy.

Yeast can be present in the vagina without causing symptoms (about 25 percent of women have yeast in their vagina at the end of their pregnancy). If it isn't causing bothersome symptoms, it doesn't need to be treated.

Yeast present in the vagina during labor will not harm the baby. Babies may develop a yeast rash in their diaper area or patches of yeast in their mouths, called thrush. These are minor problems that are easily treated. There is no evidence that treating yeast in the mother's vagina during pregnancy reduces the chance of the baby developing either of these problems.

Leg Cramps

Leg cramps (sometimes called "charley horses") are more common during pregnancy. Brenda remembers, "I woke up in the night with this terrible, really painful cramp in my leg, and I starting pounding on Marc's chest to get him to help me. He massaged my leg for a few minutes and it went away, but it happened again the next night."

Almost 50 percent of women experience these severe cramps in their leg muscles, usually at night, at some point in their pregnancy. The muscle spasm usually can be stopped by jumping quickly out of bed and standing on the leg. (Of course, this requires you to roll yourself and your pregnant belly out of bed and stand up while in considerable pain.) Massaging also seems to help.

We don't know what causes these leg cramps, or how to prevent them. The treatment most often recommended in the past was to take more calcium, but studies of calcium supplements for leg cramps during pregnancy have not found them to be any more effective than a placebo. Stretching the leg muscles for a few minutes before going to bed has been suggested as another way of preventing leg cramps, but this has not been carefully researched.

Swelling of the Legs

Swelling (edema) of the feet and legs is a common and normal symptom that at least half of women notice by the end of their pregnancy. It is caused by the normal retention of fluid by the body during pregnancy to increase the circulating blood volume. A lot of the retained fluid accumulates in the legs because of gravity, and the pressure of the uterus slows down the return of fluid to the upper body. This explains why women often notice that their hands and face are puffy when they wake up but their ankles are better, and then by the end of the day their feet and ankles are swollen once again.

Swelling requires no treatment, and there does not seem to be any treatment that is very helpful. Bed rest reduces swelling, but is rarely very practical. Keeping your feet up as much as possible can help—some women who work at desks all day may be able to rest their feet on another chair, at least some of the time. If your job requires you to be on your feet most of the day, try to sit or lie with your feet elevated during breaks.

You will feel more comfortable if you wear loose-fitting shoes—perhaps a pair in a larger size to wear at the end of the day would be useful.

> ### The Evidence About...
> ### DISCOMFORTS DURING PREGNANCY
>
> **Some of these "discomforts" can be very unpleasant for the women experiencing them, yet potential treatments have not been researched very widely. Pregnancy symptoms are common (the person who finds a prevention for stretch marks stands to make a fortune!). At present, women need to rely on trial and error to find something that eases their discomfort, and it is quite possible that many of the remedies used are no better than a placebo.**

Swelling also seems to be made worse by heat. Tanya noticed that she had much more swelling during her two summer pregnancies than when she was pregnant during the winter. "I also found that being in air-conditioned spaces really helped," she says.

Women worry about swelling because they know that it can be a symptom of pre-eclampsia, a serious disease sometimes seen in late pregnancy. Pre-eclampsia, though, also includes high blood pressure and protein in the urine—this is not normal and does require careful attention. But swelling by itself is a normal, though unpleasant, symptom of pregnancy.

Hemorrhoids and Varicose Veins

The fluid retention that is normal in pregnancy can also cause or make worse hemorrhoids (swollen veins around the anus) and varicose veins (usually in the legs, but sometimes seen in the vagina or vulva). Hemorrhoids are also made worse by constipation. There also seems to be an inherited tendency to both hemorrhoids and varicose veins.

Because fluid retention and pressure caused by the growing uterus are normal events, there is no particular prevention for them. Elastic stockings may give some relief from the aching caused by fluid retention and varicose veins in the legs, but this has never been studied.

If hemorrhoids cause no symptoms, there is no reason to treat them. If they are itchy or sore, over-the-counter hemorrhoid creams or witch hazel are soothing and will not harm the mother or baby. Avoiding constipation is essential to prevent hemorrhoids from getting worse.

12

Hypertension (High Blood Pressure) and Pre-eclampsia

You've probably noticed that every prenatal appointment includes a check of your blood pressure. What exactly is being measured? There are two numbers in every blood pressure reading: one, called the systolic blood pressure (usually given as the first or top number), measures the height of the pumping action from the heart to the artery, and the other, the bottom number or diastolic blood pressure, measures the resting pressure in the artery. These are the numbers that will be written on your chart.

Hypertension, or high blood pressure, means that the blood pressure is above a level that has been designated as the top of normal. Normal blood pressure isn't a single number; it's a range. Normal systolic blood pressure ranges from 90 to 140; normal diastolic blood pressure ranges from 60 to 90. A blood pressure of 90/60 to 140/90 is considered within the normal range; higher than 140/90 will cause concern.

Why Is It Important to Have Your Blood Pressure Checked When You're Pregnant?

Between 5 and 10 percent of pregnant women develop high blood pressure during their pregnancies. This pregnancy-induced hypertension (PIH) can cause serious problems for both mother and baby, and it's most likely to show up in the third trimester.

If a pregnant woman has PIH, plus protein in her urine (called proteinuria), plus fluid retention (swelling and puffiness), the condition is called pre-eclampsia (or toxemia, although this term is rarely used now). Pre-eclampsia rarely occurs before the third trimester. That is one reason why prenatal visits become more frequent at the end of pregnancy—to detect pre-eclampsia in its early stages, before it makes the mother sick.

Some women have high blood pressure before they get pregnant. These women's high blood pressure may improve somewhat in early pregnancy, but they are at higher risk of developing pre-eclampsia in the third trimester.

What Are the Risks of Pre-eclampsia?

In North America, 7 out of every 1000 babies die before birth. When mothers have moderate pre-eclampsia (with a diastolic pressure of 94 to 105), the risk of the baby dying triples to 21 per 1000. If the woman's blood pressure is higher than that, the risk to the baby also increases. Most of these babies die because the placenta separates from the wall of the uterus, or because the placenta stops nourishing the baby.

The baby's growth may also be restricted because of these placental problems caused by high blood pressure. While in the womb, the baby gets all of its nutrients through the placenta (via the umbilical cord), and a placenta with circulation problems won't provide enough nutrition for proper growth. That means the baby will be smaller than it should be for the length of time it has been growing inside the uterus, a condition called intra-uterine growth restriction, and it is more likely to have health problems after it is born.

Pre-eclampsia or toxemia can also be dangerous for the mother. She may have seizures (this is then called eclampsia), which can be accompanied by bleeding in the brain. The mother may even go into a coma. This condition can be fatal. The seizures can happen during pregnancy, during labor or in the 48 hours after the baby is born. Fortunately, they only happen in about 1 out of every 2000 births.

Women with severe high blood pressure can also develop kidney failure, bleeding from the liver and abnormalities of their blood-clotting mechanisms. All of these complications to the mother have been reduced with modern treatment.

What Causes Pre-eclampsia?

The cause of pre-eclampsia is unknown. It appears to be a disease that starts in the tiny blood vessels in the kidney. The underlying process probably starts months before the actual signs of elevated blood pressure and proteinuria appear.

However, there are factors that make women more likely to develop pre-eclampsia:

- first pregnancy;
- multiple pregnancy (twins, triplets, etc.);
- mother's age at pregnancy is under 18 years or over 35 years;
- mother has diabetes before becoming pregnant;
- mother has high blood pressure before becoming pregnant.

How do you know if you have pre-eclampsia? In the early stages, there are no symptoms. This is one reason why prenatal visits to your doctor or midwife are so important. Your caregiver will check your blood pressure and test your urine for protein at every visit. Towards the end of your pregnancy (when the chances of developing hypertension are higher) you will see your caregiver more frequently, so that the condition can be quickly caught if it does develop.

Many pregnant women worry about swelling or fluid retention (also called edema) because they know it is a symptom associated with pre-eclampsia. But more than half of all pregnant women will have some swelling during pregnancy, and it is perfectly normal. Unless your caregiver also finds protein in your urine and high blood pressure, you do not need to be concerned about swelling. However, swelling that occurs suddenly during pregnancy should prompt more frequent prenatal visits to check the blood pressure and urine for protein.

When pre-eclampsia begins, the expectant mother feels fine; by the time she starts to feel ill, the disease is usually severe. Some signs that the situation is very serious include headaches, pain in the upper abdomen, vomiting, blurred vision or seeing flashing lights. Any of these symptoms mean you should seek immediate medical care.

One of the frightening things about toxemia is that it is unpredictable and can progress very rapidly. Some women with mild pre-eclampsia will not get worse, and will reach the end of pregnancy with no problems for mother or baby. In other cases, a woman will have slightly elevated blood pressure and a small amount of protein in her urine one day (and be wondering what her caregiver is fussing about since she feels great). Three days later she may be feeling terrible, with severe headache, extreme swelling and dangerously high blood pressure. At present, we can't predict which cases will end up being a minor "blip" in an otherwise normal pregnancy, and which ones will end up as a serious situation.

Can Pre-eclampsia Be Prevented?

Because pre-eclampsia is a relatively common and potentially serious problem, there is great interest in methods that might prevent its development.

Diet

Many attempts have been made to reduce pre-eclampsia by modifying the diets of pregnant women. A low-salt diet was often recommended, mostly because people who eat a lot of salt tend to retain more fluid. Since there is also fluid retention involved in pre-eclampsia, the theory was that less salt might be helpful in preventing the condition. The theory doesn't hold up, though, as studies have shown that restricting salt will not prevent pre-eclampsia.

Women have also been advised to "keep their weight down" to avoid pre-eclampsia. There is no evidence that lower weight gain during pregnancy reduces the incidence of pre-eclampsia. Neither is there any evidence that increasing protein intake prevents pre-eclampsia.

A recent large study of calcium supplementation during pregnancy found that it did not reduce the risk of high blood pressure.

In short, nothing diet-related, *including* exceptionally good nutrition, has been shown to reduce the risk of pre-eclampsia.

Drugs

Various medications have also been tried, with the hope that they might prevent pre-eclampsia.

Diuretics increase the amount of urine output and reduce fluid retention. Giving diuretics to pregnant women in the hope of preventing pre-eclampsia does not work.

Some early studies suggested that low doses of aspirin might reduce the risk of pre-eclampsia in women who were at a high risk. Unfortunately, more recent, carefully designed studies have shown no benefit from aspirin.

Some women start pregnancy knowing they have had high blood pressure readings in the past. These women have a higher risk of pre-eclampsia. Doctors hoped that treating these women with high blood pressure medicine (antihypertensives) early in pregnancy, before their blood pressure got higher, would prevent the more serious symptoms of pre-eclampsia. But results have been disappointing and the medication does not seem to reduce their risk of developing severe pre-eclampsia. Similarly, women who were on blood pressure medication before becoming pregnant do not seem to be able to avoid developing pre-eclampsia by continuing their blood pressure medication in

Holly's Experience with Pregnancy-Induced Hypertension

The first six months of my pregnancy were medically uneventful. At the start of my last trimester my blood pressure started to rise a little bit. My doctor advised me that it wasn't anything to worry about, as long as it didn't get any higher and no other symptoms developed. By my 32nd week, my blood pressure was a little higher and the swelling started.

By week 33, my blood pressure and weight were still climbing and my fingers and toes looked like little pork sausages. I took a leave of absence from work and rested a lot; my blood pressure didn't improve much, but at least it didn't get worse. My 36-week visit to the doctor's office was spent talking about the possible need to be induced. I gained 40 pounds in the last few weeks of pregnancy due to edema, my blood pressure stayed up at about 150/90, but I didn't have any protein in my urine.

Sunday morning–the day before we had finally decided to induce–I woke up with labor pains. By afternoon they were about five minutes apart, so we went to the hospital.

My blood pressure had risen even higher, and I was quickly attached to a blood pressure gauge, an IV and a catheter (to measure my urine). By midnight I'd been given an epidural and oxytocin to speed up the labor. I wasn't scared, because my baby's heart rate was always good. I'll never forget the nurse who held the hand my husband wasn't holding and reassured and comforted us through a very long night. She even stayed past the shift change to see my baby born.

Because of the risk of seizures, the doctor didn't want me to push for too long. First I tried pushing myself, but I was pretty frozen from the epidural and it didn't do much. They decided to try the vacuum extractor. When it was in place, the doctor pulling on it helped me get the feeling of where to push. I pushed as hard as I could and our son, Jack, weighing 6 lbs. 6 oz., was born.

My husband was in tears. He held Jack first, and I was so happy, so tired and so relieved that I couldn't stop crying.

early pregnancy. These studies, though, have all been small.

How Is Pre-eclampsia Treated?

Once pre-eclampsia develops, delivery of the baby is the only cure. All other treatments only buy time. Of course, buying time is sometimes an important and valuable goal. If the baby is very premature, a little longer time inside the uterus will give it a better chance for survival. If pre-eclampsia is mild and the pregnancy is full-term, the extra time might allow labor to start spontaneously, avoiding induction. When

a woman is very ill with severe pre-eclampsia, the treatments described below possibly can reduce the risk of other complications and help her feel better while arrangements are made to get her baby delivered.

Common Treatments for Pre-eclampsia

Bed rest traditionally has been ordered for the mother who has pre-eclampsia. Often the mother is admitted to hospital. There is no evidence to suggest that strict bed rest, either at home or in hospital, improves any of the complications of pre-eclampsia.

However, being admitted to hospital can be useful. It allows the medical caregivers to closely monitor the mother's blood pressure and the protein levels in her urine, to perform blood tests and to assess the condition of the baby in a disease that can change rapidly. If the mother or baby is thought to be getting worse, delivery can be arranged quickly.

Melanie thought her pregnancy was going fine until, at her 32-week visit, her doctor found that her blood pressure was high and there was some protein in her urine. On his advice, she took a leave of absence from her job and rested at home. But when her blood pressure was even higher a week later, she was admitted to the hospital.

Melanie says, "I wasn't very pleased about being in the hospital, especially because I didn't feel too bad at first. Things got rapidly worse, though, and within a week I was feeling awful. I couldn't believe how swollen I was. I woke up every morning with a headache, and I was having stomachaches as well. My husband and I were really worried about the baby—I was having a non-stress test every day [a recording of the baby's heartbeat for 20 minutes]. I realized that I was going to be giving birth sooner rather than later."

Soon after that, Melanie's doctor recommended inducing labor. Although her baby girl weighed only three pounds when she was born, she was healthy and gained weight rapidly after her birth. Melanie also recovered rapidly once the baby was born, and is pleased that she has been able to successfully breast-feed her daughter despite their challenging beginning.

Antihypertensive drugs (drugs that lower blood pressure) given to a mother with pre-eclampsia can substantially reduce the risk of her already high blood pressure becoming higher. Keeping the blood pressure under control benefits the *mother* by reducing her risk of kidney damage, liver damage and brain hemorrhage. It also may reduce her chances of being induced and of having a Caesarean section.

Unfortunately, there is no good evidence that these antihypertensive drugs benefit the *baby*. They don't seem to reduce the number of stillborn babies or the number of babies with intra-uterine growth restriction. This may mean one of three things: that there really is no benefit; that the studies done so far have been too small to show any benefits; or that the benefits to some babies are outweighed by the risks to others.

Anticonvulsants are drugs that are used to prevent seizures. Once a seizure occurs, further seizures must be prevented as quickly as possible. Magnesium sulphate has been shown to be both safe and effective.

If the mother has severe pre-eclampsia, but has not yet had a seizure, doctors will often suggest one of these anticonvulsants to prevent seizures from starting. In these cases it is difficult to weigh the benefits to the mother against the risk to the baby. How severe should the pre-eclampsia be before anticonvulsants are given? How soon after this treatment will the baby be born, and how will the drug affect the baby?

Delivering the Baby

With severe pre-eclampsia and eclampsia, the best treatment is to deliver the baby.

Usually, labor is induced and the mother is kept on medication to lower her blood pressure and prevent seizures during labor. The medications will be continued for 48 hours after the baby is born. By that point, her blood pressure should be returning to normal and the risk of seizures is almost zero.

If attempts to induce labor fail, or if the woman's cervix has not begun to thin out or show any signs of readiness for labor, a Caesarean section will probably be recommended.

The Evidence About...
HYPERTENSION DURING PREGNANCY

Hypertension during pregnancy affects from 5 to 10 percent of women. Its cause is unknown. There is no treatment that prevents it from developing.

Hypertension can cause complications for the mother, and for the baby.

Pre-eclampsia (hypertension, protein in the urine and swelling) can be helped to a certain extent with medication, but the only cure is delivery of the baby.

With less severe pre-eclampsia, deciding when to induce labor is a difficult clinical judgment that worries even experienced obstetricians. This condition is fairly unpredictable and each case has to be considered individually. Even if medical treatment has produced some improvement in the blood pressure readings, the baby is still at risk. The doctor must try to decide when the risks to the baby of being premature are outweighed by the risks of the pre-eclampsia getting worse. If the cervix seems not ready for induction or if the induction doesn't work, the doctor must consider whether the risks of a Caesarean section are outweighed by the risks of the mother developing eclampsia.

13

Infections During Pregnancy

This chapter describes a number of infections that can have an impact on your pregnancy, and explains the research on their diagnosis and treatment:

- Urinary tract infections
- Chickenpox
- German measles (rubella)
- Toxoplasmosis
- Beta strep (group B streptococcus)
- Sexually transmitted diseases:
    Hepatitis B
    Herpes simplex Type Two
    AIDS
    Gonorrhea
    Chlamydia
    Syphilis

You can get infections when you are pregnant just as when you are not pregnant, but of course there are some extra concerns when a growing fetus is involved. Mothers worry about whether the infection they have will hurt the baby, and also whether the treatment could be harmful to the baby.

A woman's immune system responds to infection equally well whether she is pregnant or not. A fetus or newborn baby, though, does not handle infection as well as older children or adults. The infant's immune system is not fully functioning during its time in the uterus, or immediately after birth. The premature infant is particularly susceptible to infection.

For some infections, such as HIV and hepatitis B, there is treatment that is of clear benefit to the baby; however, this treatment cannot be given if the mother doesn't know she has the infection. A big question in pregnancy care is whether prenatal testing for these infections should be routine for all women, so that women carrying these germs can be identified and their babies can benefit from treatment.

Urinary Tract Infections (UTIs)

Wendy got a call from her doctor's nurse a few days after her first pregnancy appointment. "You've got an infection in your urine. The doctor wants you to take an antibiotic to clear it up."

Wendy was puzzled and unhappy. "But I feel fine. I really don't want to take any drugs while I'm pregnant."

"Well, your urine culture definitely shows infection—you'd better come in and talk to the doctor."

Wendy went back to the office later that week, and explained to her doctor that she felt fine and would prefer to avoid taking medication.

Her doctor responded, "I understand that you don't feel any burning or pain when going to the bathroom, but your urine culture definitely shows lots of bacteria. If you take antibiotics to clear them up now, they won't make you really sick with a bladder or kidney infection later in the pregnancy."

"Can this infection hurt my baby?" Wendy asked. "I really don't want to take any drugs in this pregnancy unless I absolutely have to."

"No, the baby's not at risk," said the doctor. "The bacteria in your urine can't affect your baby's development, the way German measles or drugs such as thalidomide can. They can just make *you* sick, sometimes really sick. And there is a very small chance that this kind of infection will start premature labor." Since Wendy was still reluctant to take antibiotics, her doctor suggested they repeat the test on her urine to be sure it was accurate.

Forty-eight hours later, Wendy got another call from her doctor: "The second culture shows exactly the same results. I think you should take the antibiotics."

What does the research say about Wendy's risks in this situation?

Three to eight percent of pregnant women have significant numbers of bacteria in their urine, without being ill or having any symptoms. This is called "asymptomatic bacteriuria" (urine bacteria). Women with urine bacteria, despite having no symptoms, have a higher chance of becoming ill with a urinary tract infection during the pregnancy, as well as a slightly higher chance of a premature delivery and low birth weight baby. The treatment of bacteria in the urine with antibiotics, even when there are no symptoms, reduces the risk of the mother becoming ill with bladder or kidney infection during the pregnancy by about 50 percent. Treatment with antibiotics also reduces the risk of premature delivery.

A number of effective antibiotics are available that are safe for use in pregnancy. The length of time needed for treatment is uncertain—continuous therapy until delivery, seven to ten days of therapy, and three days of therapy have all been equally effective.

But Wendy decided not to take antibiotics for her urine bacteria. "I drank tons of water every day and kept my bladder really flushed out. I didn't get any signs of infection ever. If I had gotten sick, then I would have taken the antibiotics. I don't think my doctor was too pleased about my decision, but it was right for me."

Bladder Infections

The woman with a bladder infection and the woman with urine bacteria have the same urine culture results. But they don't feel the same. The woman with urine bacteria feels fine—she wouldn't know she has an infection. The woman with acute cystitis (a bladder infection) feels miserable!

Urinary tract infections are common in pregnant women. One to three percent of women will have either a bladder infection or a kidney infection (pyelonephritis) during pregnancy. Drinking lots of water seems to help prevent them.

The symptoms of a bladder infection are frequent or urgent urination, burning pain when you urinate and bloody or cloudy urine. You may have all or just some of these symptoms. Frequent urination by itself is a normal part of being pregnant and not a sign of infection.

Treating bladder infections with the appropriate antibiotic relieves the symptoms of burning and frequent urination, and probably reduces the chances of it developing into a more serious kidney infection. Studies suggest that three-day treatment in pregnancy may be as effective as taking antibiotics for a longer period of time, but the data are too skimpy to make firm recommendations.

Kidney Infections

Kidney infections are, like bladder infections, more common in pregnant than non-pregnant women. This is because the collecting system of the kidney and the tubes leading from the kidneys to the bladder become wider during pregnancy. This dilation lets urine sit longer and allows bacteria to multiply.

Women with kidney infections are often acutely ill. If you have a kidney infection, you may feel pain when you urinate for a couple of days before more severe symptoms develop, but not all women experience this. When the kidney infection flares up, you will have pain in your back or side, a fever and cloudy or bloody urine. Admission to hospital for intravenous antibiotics for 48 hours is the usual treatment, with a switch to antibiotics taken orally after that.

Recent studies suggest that if the woman is not vomiting and can keep medication and fluids down, treatment with oral antibiotics is just as effective as intravenous antibiotics. Because an intravenous is not required, hospitalization may not be required either—as long as the woman is able to get the rest and care her illness requires.

About 30 percent of women who are treated

The Evidence About…
BLADDER AND KIDNEY INFECTIONS

One to three percent of women will become ill with a bladder or kidney infection sometime during their pregnancy. These can be effectively treated with antibiotics.

The treatment of bacteria in the urine with antibiotics, even when there are no symptoms, reduces the risk of the mother subsequently becoming ill with a bladder or kidney infection during the pregnancy by about 50 percent.

---

for a kidney infection during pregnancy will get another kidney infection during the same pregnancy. To try to prevent recurrence, studies have compared taking antibiotics every day until the end of the pregnancy with having regular urine cultures followed by antibiotic treatment if any bacteria are found. Both of these strategies reduce the risk of repeated kidney infections equally to about 8 percent.

The bacteria that infect the bladder and kidneys do not cause infection or illness in the fetus or newborn, except in the case of beta strep (see discussion on p. 94).

Chickenpox (Varicella-Zoster Virus)

"Chickenpox? Isn't that something children get?" Maria was shocked when the doctor diagnosed the rash of spots on her shoulders and chest.

"Usually. But clearly you didn't have it as a child, or you wouldn't have it now," he said.

Maria thought back. She didn't actually remember ever having chickenpox. "Is it dangerous to have it now, while I'm pregnant?"

When mothers get chickenpox in the first 20 weeks of pregnancy, there is a small risk (about 1.5 to 2 percent) of the baby being affected and developing abnormally.

Varicella-zoster immune globulin is a blood product given by injection to prevent chickenpox from developing after exposure to it. This immune globulin theoretically could be given to women who have been exposed to chickenpox in the first 20 weeks of pregnancy, to prevent them from developing the disease. It is rarely done, though, because the globulin has to be given within three or four days of exposure to chickenpox to be effective—and most women don't realize they have been exposed until they start to develop symptoms, usually two to three weeks later. Also, 90 percent of adults are already immune to chickenpox (even though some of them had the disease in such a mild form that they didn't know they had it).

If the mother gets chickenpox at the very end of her pregnancy, so that the baby is born while she still has the infection, it's possible for the baby to get a severe form of chickenpox and become very sick. To prevent this, a baby born to a mother with chickenpox can be given varicella-zoster immune globulin, which contains antibodies to help the baby fight the chickenpox infection.

Fortunately, Maria was seven months pregnant. At this stage of pregnancy, the chickenpox might make her a bit miserable and itchy, but it wasn't likely to cause any serious problems for her or her baby.

Rubella (German Measles)

Rubella is a virus infection that causes a mild illness—a fever and a rash—in children and

---

> ### The Evidence About...
> ### CHICKENPOX
>
> **Most women are already immune to chickenpox, but if a pregnant woman does catch it, the risks to her baby depend on how far along she is in the pregnancy.**
>
> **In the first 20 weeks chickenpox can cause birth defects in 1.5 to 2 percent of babies.**
>
> **If the mother has chickenpox at the time of delivery, it can cause a serious infection in the baby. This can be prevented by treating the baby with varicella-zoster immune globulin after it is born.**

---

adults. About a quarter of the cases show no symptoms at all. Because it is very contagious, most people catch rubella in childhood, and after that are immune to it. Rubella infection gives immunity for life. While it is a minor disease for most people, in early pregnancy it can be very serious. The rubella virus is teratogenic, meaning that it causes the fetus to develop abnormally.

The earlier in the pregnancy that the infection develops, the more serious the consequences to the fetus. *Eighty percent of women who catch rubella in the first three months of pregnancy will either miscarry or have a baby with birth defects* (called congenital rubella syndrome). After four months of pregnancy, rubella does not seem to cause any problems.

Congenital rubella syndrome is serious—babies have significant problems such as blindness and deafness. They also carry the virus in their bodies and can pass it on to other babies and to adults. There is no treatment; rubella is a virus and is not killed by antibiotics.

Rubella can, however, be prevented through vaccination. If all women were immunized against rubella before they became pregnant, congenital rubella syndrome would be eliminated. In Canada, this vaccination is recommended for all children at 13 to 14 months, with a second dose at five years of age. This is an extremely safe vaccine; in rare cases it causes a slight fever, rash and temporary joint pain.

Women who are thinking about getting pregnant can have their blood checked to see if they are immune to rubella; if they are not, they can have the rubella vaccine before they become pregnant (it takes about three months to be sure the antibodies have developed). At the first prenatal visit (as early as possible in pregnancy), blood testing for rubella antibodies is usually done. If rubella antibodies are present, there is no concern about exposure to rubella during pregnancy.

Rubella vaccine is not recommended for pregnant women, but when it has been given accidentally, none of the infants developed congenital rubella syndrome. If a pregnant woman is not immune to rubella, rubella vaccine can be given right after the baby is born, to prevent the disease in any future pregnancies. The vaccine is safe for breastfeeding mothers and their babies.

Ellen remembers: "I was sure I must have had German measles; I certainly seemed to have had everything else that was going around when I was a kid. But when they tested my blood at my first prenatal appointment, it came back negative. That had me worried—I'm a teacher, and I was terrified that I might catch it from one of the kids in my class."

Fortunately, Ellen didn't get the infection, and she arranged to be vaccinated as soon as her baby was born. "I'm glad I don't have to worry about catching German measles during this pregnancy."

While the names are similar, red measles

> ### The Evidence About...
> ### RUBELLA
>
> **The rubella virus can cause miscarriage or birth defects if caught in the early months of pregnancy. The disease cannot be treated but can be prevented by vaccination.**

(rubeola) is not the same as German measles. The red measles virus makes children and adults much sicker than rubella, and there is a vaccine against it as well, but red measles does not cause birth defects.

Toxoplasmosis

Toxoplasmosis is an infection caused by a parasite called toxoplasma gondii. It can't be passed from one person to another; instead, it is caught by eating the parasite, which is found in raw or undercooked meat or in cat feces. If, for example, you clean your cat's litter box, wash your hands less than thoroughly and then pick up some food with your fingers and eat it, it is possible (disgusting as it sounds) to have small particles of cat feces transferred to your food. You can't catch toxoplasmosis just by petting or picking up a cat.

In adults, toxoplasmosis is a mild illness, like having the flu. If you have it once, you become immune to it for life (like rubella). If you catch it during pregnancy, though, toxoplasmosis can be passed to the baby and cause serious birth defects.

When mothers get toxoplasmosis in the first three months of pregnancy, about 10 to 15 percent of babies are affected. Infected babies will usually have small heads, developmental delays, seizures and sometimes liver problems.

> ### The Evidence About . . .
> ### TOXOPLASMOSIS
>
> **Pregnant women**
>
> - **should not eat raw or undercooked meat;**
> - **should wash their hands thoroughly after handling raw meat;**
> - **should wear gloves if handling cat litter or working in a garden where cats may have been, and should wash their hands thoroughly afterwards.**

If the mother develops toxoplasmosis later in pregnancy—after six months—the baby is much more likely to be affected (60 percent risk). However, the effects at this stage are less severe. The baby may seem normal at birth, but later in childhood may develop an eye condition called chorioretinitis, which can cause blindness.

In Europe, antibiotics are now being used to treat toxoplasmosis, and there is some evidence that this is effective.

Beta Strep (Group B Streptococcus)

It might surprise you to know that all of us, even when we're perfectly healthy, have bacteria living in our bodies. We tend to think of bacteria as causing diseases, but many exist in our bodies without causing any harm to us. These bacteria are called "the normal flora," and parts of our bodies (such as the throat, bowel and vagina) will have (or "be colonized with") these normal flora most of the time.

One common and "normal" bacterium that is particularly significant for pregnant women is group B streptococcus, also called beta strep. The normal flora of a woman's vagina and rectum can include group B streptococcus. At the time of delivery, about 15 to 20 percent of women will have group B strep colonizing their vaginas.

Group B strep *usually* causes no symptoms in the mother. Occasionally, it can cause urinary tract infections, or in rare cases, an infection of the placenta, which can cause premature rupture of the membranes and premature labor.

The main reason health care professionals are concerned about this bacteria, though, is that group B strep can make newborn babies very ill. It is the most common infection in newborns. The bacteria can infect the baby during labor, or during delivery as the baby passes through the vagina.

As mentioned earlier, 15 to 20 percent of mothers carry group B strep in their vaginas during labor. Between 40 and 70 percent of the babies born to these women will be colonized with group B strep at birth. Of those "colonized" babies, only 1 to 2 percent will actually develop an infection. When you calculate all of these numbers, the rate of group B streptococcus infection in newborns is about 2 cases per 1000 babies. So even though about 20 percent of women carry these bacteria in their vaginas at the time of delivery, very few babies will be sick. Those numbers are low, but because the infection is very serious, it is still a cause for concern.

Group B strep disease in the newborn can be obvious at birth, or it can develop during the first week of life. (There is also a "late onset" group B strep disease that begins within the first three months of life and is probably caused by bacteria passed to the baby after birth. It can best be prevented by having people wash their hands thoroughly before they touch the baby.) The early onset form of this disease has generated the most attempts at prevention.

When the disease was first recognized in the 1970s, death rates were as high as 50 percent. Today the death rate is down to 10 percent. This improvement may be because the bacteria have become weaker over time, or because of earlier and more aggressive treatment. But a 10 percent death rate is still very frightening to parents with a sick baby.

When one or more of the risk factors is present (see box), the baby may be labeled "high risk" for having a strep infection. Remember that "high risk," in medical and statistical terms, means a risk significantly above the usual or normal risk. A chance of infection of 20 per 1000 when the usual rate is only 2 per 1000 would be called "high risk." But this is still an infection rate of only 2 percent; 98 percent of these babies are *not* going to be infected. So even in a group of babies labeled high risk, the majority are still not going to have a strep infection. This is important to know, because often women who are told their babies are at "high risk" of this infection think it means the baby is almost certain to be sick.

Tina's second baby had been sick with a beta strep infection but recovered and was fine. "When I got pregnant this time," Tina says, "I was told that this baby was at high risk for beta strep. I remembered how terrible it was when Zachary was sick, and I didn't know how I would go through it again. Then I went into labor prematurely—another risk factor. Mario and I were so worried. The doctor recommended intravenous antibiotics, which I had. Chloe weighed 4 lbs. 6 oz., but she never came down with beta strep. It seemed like a miracle the day we took our healthy daughter home from the hospital."

Who Is More Likely to Get Group B Strep?

Which babies are at the greatest risk of getting group B strep infection? Major risk factors include:

- baby was premature and had a low birth weight;
- membranes were ruptured for more than 18 hours before the baby was born;
- labor was long, with many interventions and frequent vaginal examinations;
- tests of mother's vagina showed heavy colonization of group B strep;
- during labor, the mother had a fever or the baby had an unusually fast heart rate;
- baby needed resuscitation at birth;
- mother has had a previous baby with a group B strep infection.

Strategies to Prevent Group B Strep

Can group B strep infections in newborns be prevented? No single strategy has been completely successful, and some treatments have been shown in clinical trials to be ineffective.

SCREENING DURING PREGNANCY

The first approach was to test all pregnant women to find out if they had group B strep in their vaginas. The test is easy and painless; the opening of the vagina is wiped with a cotton swab, which is put into culture medium in a tube and sent to the lab. It takes 24 hours to get the results.

However, colonization of the vagina by strep occurs intermittently during the nine months of pregnancy. Sometimes it's there, sometimes it's not. Seventy percent of women who tested positive for group B strep in their vaginas at 28 weeks of pregnancy did not have strep bacteria present when they were re-tested during labor.

Positive test results after 34 weeks of pregnancy are much more likely to also be positive at delivery. Testing later in pregnancy, then, sounds like a better approach. But remember the list of risk factors? A premature baby was first on the list. Waiting until after 34 weeks to do the culture means that women who go into premature labor (when the risk of infection is higher) will not have been tested, and will not know if they have group B strep in their vagina.

PREVENTIVE TREATMENT
DURING PREGNANCY

Once women with group B strep in their vaginas were identified, researchers hoped that giving these women antibiotics during pregnancy would reduce the number of babies born with the infection. Unfortunately, the studies found that this didn't work.

If the mother has a bladder infection caused by group B strep, giving antibiotics *can* be useful, as studies have shown that this reduces the chance of premature rupture of the membranes and premature labor.

PREVENTIVE TREATMENT
DURING LABOR

Although antibiotics given during pregnancy were not effective, treatment of the mother with intravenous antibiotics during labor has been shown to reduce infection rates in newborns. This is very encouraging, but leads to another question: Which women should be given the antibiotics?

The obvious solution would be to test women for beta strep during labor. However, since testing for group B strep takes at least 24 hours (longer if a lab is not constantly available), the results of tests done during labor are not available quickly enough to be useful.

Several different approaches have been suggested and are used by various caregivers:

- Testing all women for beta strep bacteria at 28 weeks of pregnancy, and treating all strep carriers who have any other risks (for example, prematurity, fever during labor, prolonged rupture of membranes) with intravenous antibiotics during labor.
- Treating all women in premature labor with IV antibiotics; and testing everyone else at 36 weeks of pregnancy and treating only those women who tested positive with intravenous antibiotics during labor.
- Treating all women who have one or more risk factors for beta strep infection, without doing any tests for strep.

Each of these approaches has been shown to reduce the risk of newborn strep infection. Unfortunately, though, each of these approaches also means giving antibiotics to many, many women whose babies would never have developed an infection anyway.

TREATING THE BABY AFTER BIRTH

Newborns with group B strep infections are born with the illness already present, or become ill in the first few hours after birth. But the symptoms are not very obvious.

If your baby is born infected with group B strep, his early symptoms will be vague: he could be lethargic, irritable and not feeding well. He may have fast heart and respiration rates. Cultures of the baby's blood and spinal fluid are the definitive way to make the diagnosis, but it takes 24 to 48 hours to get results. It's important to diagnose this infection quickly, because the earlier the baby is treated with antibiotics, the better the outcome.

This puts the doctor, and the parents, in a difficult position. Is newborn baby Adam lethargic, or just a relaxed and quiet baby? Is

The Evidence About...
BETA STREP

This is a rare (2 cases per 1000 babies) but serious infection for newborn babies.

While some risk factors are known, we can't predict very accurately which babies will develop the problem. Any treatment to reduce the number of infected babies will mean giving antibiotics to large numbers of mothers and babies who don't need them, and will miss some babies who really do need treatment.

The side-effects of this treatment may seem minor for the individual mother and baby, but the consequences of increasingly resistant bacteria are serious for our society as a whole.

baby Bethany jittery and irritable because of illness or because she has a sensitive and fussy temperament? How long should the doctor wait before starting treatment? Most pediatricians feel "it's better to be safe than sorry," so many infants who do not have infections are treated with antibiotics to be sure that the few who are infected are treated early.

Some infants will be born looking perfectly well, but considered to be at risk for infection because of one or more risk factors during labor, such as a mother colonized by strep, prolonged rupture of the membranes or prematurity. There are no good studies to suggest the best way to take care of these babies. Routines for their care will vary from hospital to hospital, and even among individual pediatricians at the same hospital. These routines include:

- The usual care given to every baby, with no special tests or antibiotics.
- Doing blood counts and cultures for strep, and then observing the baby while waiting for these results.
- Giving preventive intravenous antibiotics, for varying lengths of time, without waiting for the results of tests or observations.

There are no studies to suggest which of these approaches is the best care for babies who look well but are identified as being at risk. Similarly, there are no studies to suggest the best care for babies whose mothers have received antibiotics during labor because of risk factors, but who are born looking perfectly well. Since there isn't any conclusive research, you and your doctor should evaluate your individual situation and make a decision together about the best approach.

Overuse of Antibiotics: Why the Concern?

Does it matter that antibiotics are being given to many mothers and babies who would never develop this disease?

Yes, because there are side-effects and complications from antibiotics that are significant. The most important complication of unnecessary antibiotic use is the development of resistant bacteria—bacteria that do not die when the sick person is given antibiotics. (It is the bacteria that become resistant, not the person.) This is an increasingly serious problem in our society, but it does not affect, in any way we can measure, the individual mother and her baby at the time she is given the antibiotics.

For individual mothers and babies, antibiotics can cause side-effects such as diarrhea and yeast infections. There is also an effect, difficult to measure, of labeling babies as "high risk" and separating them from their mothers to treat them with IV antibiotics. This creates anxiety in the mother, may make it difficult to establish breastfeeding and may affect the relationship she develops with her baby.

Regina's premature baby was considered to be at high risk of infection and was treated with antibiotics in the intensive care nursery. Regina was discharged from the hospital and had to leave her newborn behind, although she visited every day. Regina remembers: "I think it was worse for my husband Alec than it was for me. I spent more time with the baby, and I thought he looked pretty good. But my husband focused on the IV and the monitoring equipment and how small our son was, and he was convinced he was going to die." Even when the baby came home, Alec felt nervous handling the baby and Regina says it took him some time to believe that this child would survive.

Sexually Transmitted Diseases (STDs)

There are infections that are passed from one person to another during sexual activity. It can be embarrassing to discuss these diseases with your doctor, yet diagnosis is important because some have significant effects on your unborn baby and can be treated.

Screening for Sexually Transmitted Diseases

STDs such as syphilis, herpes, AIDS and hepatitis B are common in our society, and therefore are common in pregnant women. Any woman who is sexually active (and this obviously includes all pregnant women) can get an STD, but some women are more at risk than others. The more sexual partners a woman has

had, the higher her risk of coming in contact with one or more STDs.

Some other risk factors for having an STD have do with "lifestyle." Young, single and low-income women have higher STD rates. Intravenous drug use is also a risk factor. But most of the women in these groups do not have STDs, and about 40 percent of the people who have STDs don't belong to any of these groups.

Should you be tested for STDs? If you are high risk, you will probably answer "yes." But what if you are in a low-risk group? It's still possible for you to have an infection that could harm your baby, yet if all low-risk pregnant women get tested, the costs will be very high for little benefit.

Hepatitis B

Hepatitis B is a virus that affects the liver. It is passed from person to person through direct contact with blood, saliva, vaginal secretions or semen, or it can be transmitted at birth from a mother carrying the hepatitis B virus to her infant.

Ninety percent of adults infected with hepatitis B will recover completely and are then immune to the disease. Ten percent develop chronic hepatitis—they continue to carry the hepatitis B virus in their blood. These people can develop cirrhosis or liver cancer. As well, they are infectious to people with whom

Risk Factors for Sexually Transmitted Diseases

- Multiple sexual partners;
- if one sexually transmitted disease is present, the risk of others also being present is higher;
- intravenous drug use.

they have sexual relations, or with whom they share needles, or to their unborn babies.

Routine testing of large groups of women shows a positive test for hepatitis B in almost 1 percent. About 20 percent of babies born to infected mothers will catch the virus and develop chronic hepatitis. Infection usually happens during the birth when the baby comes in contact with the mother's vaginal secretions.

TREATING THE BABY EXPOSED TO HEPATITIS B

If a mother is carrying hepatitis B, her baby's risk of infection can be reduced from 20 percent to almost zero by injecting the baby with hepatitis B immune globulin as soon as it is born. This globulin contains antibodies from the blood of people already immune to hepatitis B. At the same time, the baby is given an injection of the hepatitis B vaccine, to stimulate it to make its own antibodies. Two more doses of hepatitis B vaccine are given when the baby is two months old and four months old to make the baby completely immune to hepatitis B.

The Evidence About . . .
HEPATITIS B

Hepatitis B immune globulin can protect babies born to mothers with hepatitis B from infection.

A mother can't give her baby the benefits of the hepatitis B immune globulin at birth unless she knows she is carrying the virus, so it seems reasonable for all pregnant women to get tested for hepatitis B.

If everyone was vaccinated against hepatitis B, it would protect babies from this disease.

Herpes Simplex

Herpes simplex is a virus that can be transmitted from one person to another by touch or by kissing. There are two types:

- Type One is responsible for the common "cold sore" or "fever blister" around the mouth. It can occasionally cause sores around the genitals as well.
- Type Two is often called genital herpes, because it is usually found on the genitals. It is most often caught during sexual contact. This Type Two virus is of most concern to pregnant women, because it can be passed to the baby at birth.

Herpes is very difficult to diagnose, but it is estimated that about 20 percent of women may have the herpes Type Two virus. Although this virus is very common, only a very few babies will catch the infection from their mothers. While we don't know exactly how many, estimates vary between 1 in 2500 and 1 in 10,000 babies infected.

MATERNAL HERPES TYPE TWO INFECTIONS

Many women who have herpes are not aware of it. A woman's first attack or outbreak of genital herpes is usually the most severe. Often she will have a fever, aching and tiredness, plus small, painful sores in the vaginal area. There are exceptions—some women with their first outbreak will have only small sores and no other symptoms of illness. The initial attack usually ends within one to three weeks and the sores heal without leaving any sign that they were ever there.

However, the herpes virus is not gone. It can continue to live in the body for long periods of time without causing any symptoms—this is called latent or dormant herpes. After the first attack, some women will never again have the painful open sores. Others have recurrent attacks, usually milder than the first. During these attacks, and for some days afterwards, live herpes virus is present in the vaginal area. There may also be live herpes virus present at times when the woman is not having an obvious attack, but this is rare. There is no cure for herpes.

The baby is at the highest risk of infection if the mother has her first (primary) outbreak of herpes right at the time of labor and delivery. At this point her body has not had time to develop any antibodies that would protect the baby from the infection.

When there is a primary outbreak of herpes at the beginning of labor, a Caesarean section may prevent the baby from catching the herpes virus, especially if the membranes have not ruptured. (If they have, there is a small possibility that the baby may have already picked up the virus, but usually herpes is caught as the baby passes through the birth canal.)

If the mother has had recurrent attacks of herpes, she already has antibodies that have been passed on to the baby through the placenta, so the risk to the baby is less. Studies of women with recurrent genital herpes found that only 1.4 percent had live herpes virus present during labor. If there are no open sores, the baby is at minimal risk of infection during a vaginal birth.

While herpes infections of newborn babies are not common, they are potentially serious. Since there is no cure, researchers have concentrated on ways to prevent babies from catching herpes.

Tests can be done to see if live herpes virus is present when women are in labor, but the results come back too late to be useful. Testing during late pregnancy cannot predict which mothers will be infectious at the time the baby is born.

One study compared pregnant women with

The Evidence About...
HERPES

While genital herpes is very common (about 20 percent of women may have had it), herpes infections of newborn babies are very rare (between 1 in 2500 and 1 in 10,000).

Caesarean section is currently recommended for women with active herpes outbreaks at the time they go into labor, although this is not supported by strong evidence.

---

recurrent herpes who were treated with an antiviral drug to a similar group of pregnant women who did not receive the drug. The drug significantly reduced the risk of live herpes virus being present in the vagina at the time of delivery. Because of the rareness of the infection, though, neither group had any cases of herpes infection of the newborn.

Some physicians and hospitals have recommended Caesarean sections for all women with a history of genital herpes, but there is absolutely no research to support this. The Society of Obstetricians and Gynaecologists of Canada currently recommends that, when labor begins, *Delivery by Caesarean section is only indicated in the presence of clinically active lesions (open sores) in the lower genital tract.* Even this recommendation is not strongly supported by research.

Alana was very pleased when she heard about this new recommendation during her second pregnancy. "I had a Caesarean with my first pregnancy because my doctor recommended it for all women with herpes. I was dreading the surgery and recovery when I got pregnant again, but this time I was able to have a VBAC."

CARE OF THE NEWBORN

If your baby is born when you have an outbreak of genital herpes, the baby should be isolated from other newborns—*but not from you!* Breastfeeding will benefit the baby just as it does any other baby. You will need to wash your hands carefully before touching the baby and make sure she doesn't come in contact with any of the herpes sores. The baby will be carefully watched, and can be treated with anti-herpes virus drugs if a fever, rash or other signs of illness develop.

Babies can also catch herpes Type One—the common cold sore—so anyone who has a cold sore should not kiss the baby or touch the baby without thoroughly washed hands.

AIDS

AIDS (Acquired Immunodeficiency Syndrome) is a widely publicized disease caused by HIV (Human Immunodeficiency Virus). It has become the third leading cause of death of American women between the ages of 25 and 44—the years during which most women have babies.

There is a huge amount of research currently underway on various treatments for people with AIDS. Still, at present there is no cure and the death rate is high.

No one knows exactly how many pregnant

The Evidence About...
AIDS

Treatment of the HIV positive mother and her baby with zidovudine greatly reduces the rate of HIV transmission to the baby.

If testing for HIV is only offered to high-risk groups, many women who are HIV positive will be missed, and their babies will not get the benefit of treatment.

Letting pregnant women know about zidovudine may encourage them to be tested.

---

women are HIV positive. The Center for Disease Control has estimated an overall rate of 1 to 2 per 1000, but in some communities the rate is much higher.

If a woman infected with the HIV virus becomes pregnant, she has a 13 to 40 percent chance of infecting her baby; the average rate is about 30 percent. *This rate can be dramatically reduced by treatment with the antiviral drug zidovudine.* If given to the HIV positive mother during pregnancy, and to the infant for the first six weeks after birth, it reduces the rate of HIV transmission from 30 to 8 percent.

Breastfeeding can transmit HIV from mother to baby, although the risk appears to be small. In wealthy countries, where there is sufficient formula and clean water to mix it with, formula feeding will avoid the small risk of transmission through breast milk. In developing countries, the World Health Organization still recommends breastfeeding, even if the mother is HIV positive, as the advantages of breastfeeding would outweigh the small risk of HIV transmission.

How HIV Is Transmitted

- Through sexual contact with an infected person's body fluids;
- through blood transfusions of infected blood;
- through sharing needles contaminated with infected blood;
- during pregnancy, from an infected mother to her child.

Recent research suggests that Caesarean section before the start of labor decreases still further the baby's risk of acquiring HIV from an infected mother. Unfortunately, the world populations with the highest rates of HIV infection are also the least likely to have access to safe Caesarean section.

Other Sexually Transmitted Diseases

GONORRHEA

Gonorrhea is a sexually transmitted disease caused by a bacteria called gonococcus. Some women with gonorrhea have a greenish vaginal discharge, fever and pain in the pelvic area. During pregnancy, women with gonorrhea are more likely to feel very ill, with hot, painful joints as well as fever and pelvic pain. However, many women who have gonorrhea have no symptoms at all.

Women with gonorrhea are more likely to give birth prematurely. After a miscarriage or after the birth of her baby, the mother who has gonorrhea can get a bad uterine infection that needs to be treated with antibiotics. This infection can reduce her chances of getting pregnant again by causing scar tissue that blocks the Fallopian tubes.

Gonorrhea can be tested for during a prenatal visit. If it is present, the mother can take antibiotics that are safe during pregnancy to cure the infection. The baby doesn't catch gonorrhea while it is in the uterus, but picks up the infection while it passes through the birth canal. If the mother has been treated with antibiotics, the baby is also protected.

A baby born to a mother with untreated gonorrhea is at risk of developing a serious eye infection that can cause blindness if not treated. The infection usually develops two to five days after birth. In many countries, treatment of all newborns (to kill any gonorrhea bacteria) with silver nitrate eye drops, or, more

> **The Evidence About...**
> **GONORRHEA**
>
> Routine treatment—drops or ointment in the baby's eyes shortly after birth—has been carried out to successfully prevent eye infections and blindness from gonorrhea for more than 100 years.
>
> Undiagnosed and untreated gonorrhea can cause serious infections in the mother's uterus.

recently, with antibiotic eye ointments, is required by law. The ointments are more effective in preventing eye infections from both gonorrhea and chlamydia, and are less irritating to the baby's eyes.

Researchers have compared treating all babies with these ointments soon after birth with watching to see if the infection develops and promptly treating only the infected babies. The results were equally good with both methods. However, it is difficult to observe and treat only infected babies because of the trend towards shorter hospital stays after birth. Routine treatment of all babies is the law in most places.

CHLAMYDIA

Chlamydia trachomatis is the most common sexually transmitted bacteria in women of childbearing age. Various studies have found that between 2 and 25 percent of pregnant women (this is a hard bacterium to diagnose!) have chlamydia.

Chlamydia can cause a yellow-green vaginal discharge, and can make women ill with fever and pelvic pain. However, in most women (and men), the infection causes no symptoms at all. Chlamydia is only caught during sexual intercourse, so women who have many sexual partners are more likely to come in contact with it.

How does chlamydia affect pregnancy and birth? It is suspected that chlamydia may cause premature rupture of the membranes, and premature birth of the baby, but the studies on this have been contradictory.

However, the risk of infection to the baby is clear. Between 20 and 50 percent of babies born to mothers infected with chlamydia will develop an eye infection; if this condition is not treated, it can lead to blindness. The standard eye ointment given to babies to prevent gonorrhea infections (silver nitrate, erythromycin ointment or tetracycline ointment) will prevent about 80 percent of chlamydia eye infections. If an infection does develop, the baby will need to be treated with antibiotics. Between 3 and 18 percent of babies born to infected mothers will develop chlamydia pneumonia. This can also be treated with antibiotics.

Can we prevent chlamydia infection in babies? It is difficult to diagnose chlamydia in pregnant women: tests are expensive and are not completely accurate. Treatment during pregnancy is also challenging, because the most effective drug (tetracycline) should not be used during pregnancy. A slightly less effective drug (erythromycin) tends to give women stomachaches and make them vomit, but erythromycin is considered safe during pregnancy.

One study compared women who took antibiotics for chlamydia during pregnancy with another group who chose not to be treated. The babies of the women who were treated had significantly lower rates of infection.

SYPHILIS

Syphilis is a sexually transmitted disease that can be passed from an infected mother to her baby through the placenta. In Canada and the United States, the law requires all pregnant

> ### The Evidence About...
> ### CHLAMYDIA
>
> **There is a lot of uncertainty about how common chlamydia infections are. What is certain is that the bacteria can be dangerous to newborns.**
>
> **If you are at risk of having chlamydia, you could ask to be tested. Treatment with antibiotics while you are pregnant will significantly reduce the risk to your baby.**

women to be tested for syphilis at their first prenatal visit. (Remember having all that blood taken then? Some of it was used to test for syphilis.) This test does have some false positives, but further testing will confirm whether the mother is actually infected.

However, women who have caught syphilis within the past four to six weeks will test negative, even though they actually have the disease. This false negative could be picked up if women who are at higher risk of having syphilis are tested again later in the pregnancy. Once it is diagnosed, syphilis is easily treated with penicillin.

Syphilis starts with a painless "pimple" in the genital area that heals by itself. Weeks later, there is a rash and flu-like symptoms, which also go away by themselves. During these early stages, the disease is completely curable with penicillin. If it is not treated, the disease can be dormant for many years, before causing severe damage to the heart and nervous system. During all this time, the woman is infectious to other people through sexual activity or her blood.

If a mother has syphilis and it is left untreated, her baby has an almost 100 percent chance of catching syphilis before birth. About 20 to 40 percent of these babies will die before birth. If the baby is born with congenital syphilis, it may be very ill, with permanent damage to the heart, lungs and liver. Other babies are born looking well but have syphilis germs present in the bloodstream and nervous system. All of these babies can be treated with penicillin, but, while the drug will kill the germs, it can't heal the damage that is already done.

If the mother is treated with penicillin, the cure rate for her is virtually 100 percent. The cure rate for her unborn baby depends on how long the baby was infected. Usually the fetus does not pick up the infection until after the 18th week of pregnancy, so early treatment means the baby is likely to be healthy. Later in the pregnancy, penicillin may cure the mother but may not prevent harm to the baby. About 20 percent of babies born to mothers treated for syphilis towards the end of pregnancy will have been damaged by syphilis.

Talking to Your Doctor about STDs During Pregnancy

If you feel you are at risk for a sexually transmitted disease, because of multiple sexual partners, for example, you may feel uncomfortable talking to your doctor about this issue. But the test results and treatment can make a huge difference to your baby, so it is well worth overcoming your anxiety.

Andrea struggled with asking about testing. "I'd been with quite a few men before I settled down with Quentin, and I have to confess we

---

The Evidence About . . .
SYPHILIS

A woman with syphilis may look and feel well, but the disease she is carrying, if left untreated, will be tragic for her baby. This is why the law requires every pregnant woman to be tested. Early treatment when syphilis is present can prevent serious problems for the baby as well as cure the mother.

---

didn't always use condoms. Okay, I was young and foolish. I figured I could just put my past behind me—until I got pregnant."

Andrea decided she wanted the testing done, but dreaded making the request. "I couldn't sleep all night before my doctor's appointment. What if it turned out I had AIDS? How would I tell Quentin? And I wondered how my doctor would react."

As it turned out, though, her doctor was very understanding. "I started off saying I wanted to be tested for STDs, and then I was stumbling around trying to explain why, and my doctor told me I didn't have to explain my reasons, he'd be happy to arrange for the tests to be done." To Andrea's relief, they all came back negative.

"I'm glad I did it," she says. "If it turned out I had an infection, it's better to know and be tested—especially when there's a baby involved."

14

Miscarriage and Ectopic Pregnancy

"I'm bleeding!" Carole called her doctor in a panic. "There's blood in my underpants—it looks like the start of my period."

At her first pregnancy appointment, at six weeks, everything had seemed fine. Now, just two weeks later, she was bleeding.

In the office, her doctor looked at her cervix with a speculum. The blood was definitely coming from inside the uterus. "I had hoped it might just be some irritation on your cervix bleeding, but it isn't," said her doctor. "You might be starting to miscarry."

Carole started to cry. "What can I do to stop it? I can't lose my baby."

Her doctor took her hand sympathetically. "If your baby is going to be fine, it is. If you are going to have a miscarriage, you are. There is nothing you or I can do to change that."

Carole said, "I'll go home and go to bed for a couple of days. I'll just take the time off work. I'll do anything to keep from losing my baby."

Again her doctor tried to comfort her. "Carole, I know you would do anything; I know you really want this baby. But going to bed isn't going to keep you from having a miscarriage. If you start having heavier bleeding and cramps, you might want to stay in bed for your own comfort, but it isn't going to keep you from miscarrying."

Carole called her doctor again the next day. "I'm still bleeding, sort of like a light period. I don't have any bad pain though. That's a good sign, isn't it?"

Her doctor suggested having an ultrasound to see if the baby was still alive.

Carole was upset. "How will that help? I didn't want to have any ultrasounds during my pregnancy."

Her doctor explained that having an ultrasound would tell them whether the baby was alive, but it wouldn't change the fact that there was no treatment that would help. Carole decided to wait a few more days.

That night, Carole barely slept. The bleeding was heavier and she had painful cramps. Towards morning, her husband drove her to the hospital. "I guess I'm having a miscarriage—surely I couldn't have cramps and

Did I Cause My Miscarriage?

Miscarriage is *not* caused by:

- too much exercise;
- too little exercise;
- eating junk food;
- going dancing;
- using computers or video display terminals;
- not wanting to be pregnant;
- having sex;
- whatever you did the day before you started bleeding.

You *cannot* prevent a miscarriage by:

- resting in bed;
- eating really well;
- taking estrogen or progesterone pills;
- taking vitamins or minerals or herbal supplements.

bleeding this bad and the baby still be okay," she said to her doctor when he arrived.

Her doctor examined her again. "Yes, you are having a miscarriage. There's a lot of blood and clots here now, and I think your uterus feels a little smaller than it did. I don't know what will happen from here. You may finish miscarrying and the bleeding will stop on its own. Or you may keep on bleeding and cramping for days, until you have a D&C, a dilation and curettage, to scrape out all the tissue that is left in your uterus."

Carole's doctor again suggested having an ultrasound: "It will tell for sure that you don't have a live baby. And it will also show how much tissue is left in the uterus. If there isn't much, you are probably fine just to go home and let your body handle this by itself, without having a D&C."

Carole decided to have the ultrasound: "I cried all the way through it. The technician was so business-like, and didn't say anything to me at all. My friends had told me about ultrasounds where they had seen the baby and seen its heartbeat. When I asked the technician, he said he couldn't tell me anything, I would have to ask my doctor."

The ultrasound showed no live baby, and very little tissue left in the uterus. Carole went home. She stopped bleeding about four days later, and got her normal period six weeks after that.

A miscarriage (also called a spontaneous abortion) is the death of a fetus before 20 weeks of pregnancy. Miscarriage is common—probably about 35 percent of all pregnancies end in miscarriage. About 25 percent of pregnancies miscarry before the woman even knows she is pregnant. She may think her period is just a little late, or a little heavier than usual, but in fact she did have a fertilized egg and is having an early miscarriage. Another 10 percent of pregnancies miscarry after the woman has missed her period and realizes she is pregnant. At least 85 percent of miscarriages happen before 12 weeks of pregnancy.

Causes of Miscarriage

There is probably more misinformation about the causes of miscarriage than any other area of pregnancy. Many women worry that they caused their miscarriage by having sex, moving heavy furniture or exercising too much—none of which are related to miscarriage. Often women blame whatever they did the day before the bleeding started, when in fact, the baby usually dies several days before the bleeding of miscarriage begins.

There is *no* increased association of miscarriage with bad nutrition, vigorous exercise, sedentary lifestyle, video display terminals or pregnancies that happen as a result of failures of oral contraceptives or spermicidal creams and jellies. Pregnancies that are planned and wanted miscarry just as often as pregnancies that are unwanted.

About 50 percent of miscarried fetuses have genetic problems. The miscarriage could be regarded as nature's solution to an abnormal embryo. The other 50 percent of fetuses miscarry for various reasons, many of them unknown. It may not have been a perfect egg or a perfect sperm, or perhaps the developing embryo did not implant itself in a good spot in the wall of the uterus.

There are some situations where miscarriages are more common:

- When mothers smoke, drink more than two alcoholic drinks per day or use recreational drugs, miscarriage is slightly more common.
- If the mother becomes pregnant with an IUD in place, she is more likely to miscarry.
- Women with diabetes have a higher rate of miscarriage. If the mother's blood sugar is perfectly controlled during the weeks before conception and in the early weeks of the pregnancy, this risk is reduced.
- Older mothers are slightly more likely to miscarry, because they are more likely to have babies with abnormal chromosomes.
- Infections such as German measles or syphilis in early pregnancy can cause miscarriage.

Terms Used to Discuss Miscarriage

Threatening to Miscarry

Any woman who has bleeding in early pregnancy is likely to be described as "threatening to miscarry," although that isn't very accurate. About half the women who have vaginal bleeding in early pregnancy will miscarry, but for the other half the bleeding may have nothing at all to do with miscarriage.

Rita says, "In three out of my four pregnancies, I had two or three days of bleeding about two weeks after my period was due. The first time I worried about it, but after that I thought it was normal for me. My sister had the same experience when she was pregnant—and I know this sounds weird, but for both of us it only happened when we were carrying boys."

Leslie remembers her first 10 weeks of pregnancy with anger. "I had some bleeding at six weeks and at seven weeks and at nine weeks. Each time it stopped by itself, and each time I had an ultrasound. The doctor said I was 'okay for now, we'll see how things go in the next couple of weeks.'

"Finally, when I bled again at 11 weeks, my doctor examined me and found that I had a polyp on my cervix that was bleeding. It had nothing to do with the pregnancy at all. He removed it and I never bled again. It makes me mad that I worried for 10 weeks about my baby and had three ultrasounds for nothing."

Leslie says that if she had this kind of bleeding again during pregnancy, she would insist on having it more thoroughly investigated.

Inevitable Miscarriage or Inevitable Abortion

The woman who is having heavy bleeding with clots, has leaked amniotic fluid and has a soft, open cervix is having an inevitable miscarriage. The fetus is already dead, and is in the process of being passed from the uterus.

An inevitable miscarriage may also be diagnosed by an ultrasound that shows that the baby has died or was never formed. Even though the woman may not be bleeding very heavily at that moment, she is eventually going to miscarry.

The diagnosis of inevitable miscarriage can also be made by repeating the blood test for pregnancy. If the levels of pregnancy hormone are lower than average, and are getting lower rather than higher in the first 12 weeks of pregnancy, the pregnancy is going to miscarry.

Many women who are going to miscarry will comment that they don't "feel pregnant" any more, even if they are only bleeding lightly (or sometimes not at all). This is because they are no longer producing pregnancy hormones, and they will eventually miscarry.

Mary says, "I knew something was wrong when I got up in the morning and started dressing my kids to take them to the playground. I was doing up Paul's coat when I realized that I didn't feel queasy at all. I felt normal. When I met my friend at the park, I told her I thought I was going to miscarry, because I didn't feel pregnant any more. And I was right. The bleeding started the next day."

Incomplete Miscarriage or Incomplete Abortion

This means that the miscarriage is inevitable but there is still tissue in the uterus, which may cause the woman to keep on bleeding and cramping.

Missed Abortion

This means that the fetus has died, sometimes weeks earlier, but has not been expelled from the uterus. Usually the woman doesn't feel pregnant any more, her uterus isn't growing and her breasts are back to normal, but she hasn't had the bleeding and cramping to expel the dead fetus. A missed abortion will expel itself eventually, or if it is diagnosed by ultrasound, the woman may choose to have a D&C.

Blighted Ovum

A blighted ovum is a miscarriage in which there has been a fertilized egg, but it died so early that no actual fetus has formed. An ultrasound will show a small, empty sac in the uterus with no fetus in it. Often in this situation, the woman has never felt very pregnant, but she did miss a period and have a positive pregnancy test. This miscarriage usually doesn't cause a lot of bleeding, and usually doesn't need a D&C.

Recurrent Miscarriage

A recurrent miscarriage is one that occurs in a woman who has already had a miscarriage. Many researchers have studied women who have more than one miscarriage to see if they have some common problem. To date, there seems to be nothing that these women have in common except bad luck. In some individual cases, there may be physical problems that make it more difficult for the mother to carry a baby to full term.

A small subgroup of women who have had three or more consecutive miscarriages, without ever having a full-term pregnancy, have been studied for the possibility of immunity problems between them and their partners. This research looks promising, but is as yet inconclusive.

Ultrasound and Miscarriage

Ultrasound has been extremely helpful to mothers who are concerned that they are having a miscarriage. Ultrasound can detect a fetal sac by 35 days after the last menstrual period, and a fetal heartbeat by 45 days after the last period. If the woman is unsure of her dates, sometimes two ultrasounds about a week apart are needed to distinguish a blighted ovum from a very early pregnancy.

Ultrasound can also help in decision making about the need for a D&C by showing how much tissue is left in the uterus.

Prevention of Miscarriage

There is almost as much misinformation about the prevention of miscarriage as there is about its causes. The research can be summarized quickly: *nothing* so far has been demonstrated to prevent miscarriage.

Two main approaches to preventing miscarriage have been tried: bed rest and hormones.

Bed Rest

For years, women who had any bleeding in early pregnancy were told to rest in bed. Studies have shown that women who rest in bed miscarry just as often as women who continue their usual activities. Unfortunately, bed rest continues to be advised on the basis that "it can't do any harm." This is not true; bed rest can be harmful. Women who go to bed are disrupting their lives, their households and their jobs, for no benefit. Women who don't confine themselves to bed (and how many women can?) and then miscarry often feel guilty unnecessarily, believing that if they had rested more, they could have saved their babies.

Hormone Therapy

DES (diethylstilboestrol) is a hormone that was given to women in countries all over the world for over 30 years (from the 1940s to the 1970s) in the belief that it prevented miscarriage. By the 1950s, research trials had clearly shown that it did not prevent miscarriage.

The tragic result of that unsuccessful attempt to prevent miscarriage is that children born to women who took DES during their pregnancy are at a higher risk of serious health problems (among them, infertility and vaginal cancer). What makes this truly tragic is that DES continued to be widely used for 15 years after the research had demonstrated that it didn't work to prevent miscarriage. Its use was only stopped when early reports of the harm it had done to children were made public.

Hormone treatment with progesterone-like drugs is currently being used to try to prevent miscarriage. There are good reasons to think that progesterone is needed to maintain the growth of the fetus in the first 12 to 20 weeks. To date, no studies have demonstrated the usefulness of progesterone-like drugs in preventing miscarriage, although this research is ongoing.

Tubal (Ectopic) Pregnancy

When Lesley became pregnant for the fourth time, she expected everything to go as smoothly as it had with her first three. A week after her first prenatal visit, though, she got a pain in her side, bad enough to make her call her doctor and say she needed to be seen that day. "I knew I had never felt anything like it with my other pregnancies." As soon as the doctor examined her, he sent her for an ultrasound, which showed what he had suspected: Lesley had a tubal (ectopic) pregnancy.

The father's sperm and the mother's ovum or egg normally meet and combine to start the growth of the embryo inside the mother's Fallopian tubes (these tubes run between the ovary, where the eggs are produced, and the uterus). Over the next few days, this embryo continues down the Fallopian tubes and into the uterus. There it makes a home in the uterine lining and starts developing into the fetus and placenta.

In a tubal pregnancy, the embryo doesn't make it all the way to the uterus. Instead, it grows inside the Fallopian tube. This is dangerous because although the uterus can grow very dramatically throughout pregnancy, the Fallopian tube can't. That means that soon the rapidly growing embryo will rupture the tube, causing internal bleeding and pain.

Lesley had surgery that night to remove the tubal pregnancy, and while the operation and her recovery went well, the experience was difficult emotionally. She says, "First I found out I was pregnant, and we started planning for the new baby. We were feeling excited and positive. Then the next thing I know, I'm having major surgery—and there's no baby. I was worried, too, that this would affect my chances of getting pregnant again."

Tubal pregnancies occur in about 1 pregnancy out of 100. They are more common in these situations:

- If a woman has had a previous pelvic infection that has scarred her tubes, tubal pregnancy is more likely.
- If a woman has had one ectopic pregnancy, her risk of having another is from 7 to 15 percent.
- Women who become pregnant with an IUD in place, or after a tubal ligation, are more likely to have a tubal pregnancy.
- Women who become pregnant using fertility treatments are at higher risk for tubal pregnancy.

Treatment of Tubal Pregnancy

Possibly 40 percent of tubal pregnancies will end spontaneously without the woman ever knowing she was pregnant. The fetus dies very early on and is gradually reabsorbed without the woman experiencing any pain or bleeding. Her period may be a little bit late or a little bit heavier than usual, but that is all.

When tubal pregnancy causes enough pain and bleeding to be diagnosed, it is usually treated with surgery, either through a laparoscope, which only requires a small incision in the abdomen, or through surgery with a full abdominal incision.

Another treatment has been developed recently to try to avoid surgery for tubal preg-

nancy. With this treatment, a drug called methotrexate is injected intramuscularly into the mother or through the abdominal wall into the tiny sac containing the embryo. The embryo will be reabsorbed and the mother will have a fairly heavy period, but the Fallopian tube will be saved. This works about 90 percent of the time, and is most successful when the diagnosis is made early in pregnancy. If this drug treatment is not successful, surgery will be required.

When there is surgery after a tubal pregnancy, the affected Fallopian tube is removed, which may make it more difficult for a women to get pregnant again.

Grieving after a Miscarriage

Often family or friends consider a miscarriage to be a fairly minor loss, certainly not as significant as a stillbirth or the death of a newborn. Yet for the mother, and sometimes for the father, a miscarriage can be very traumatic. Once a pregnancy is confirmed, parents may begin to make plans for the new addition to their family, and a miscarriage may be the loss of a very real baby.

Leanne says, "One day we were all excited about the baby, picking out names and planning how we'd decorate the nursery. Then the next day the bleeding started, and by Friday there was no baby. Nothing. I could hardly bring myself to leave the house—I was afraid that if I saw someone with a baby I'd just break down and cry."

Besides the physical care provided, women who have experienced a threatened or an actual miscarriage will also need emotional support.

Amanda remembers being appalled by the attitude of the emergency ward doctor who treated her miscarriage. "She told me to be grateful, that the baby probably wouldn't have

Bleeding in the Second Half of Pregnancy

"Normal show" or "bloody show" is the name given to the slight vaginal bleeding that often is the first sign that labor is starting. The blood is usually mixed with thick mucus and may be more pink than red when you see it. Any other bleeding in the latter half of pregnancy is not normal, and *should be reported to your caregiver right away.*

About half of the women who have bleeding in the second half of their pregnancy are found to have either a "placenta previa" or an "abruption of the placenta." For the other half, the cause of the bleeding is not found.

Abruption of the Placenta

This is the separation of part of the placenta from the wall of the uterus before the delivery of the baby. It can range from a minor bit of bleeding, which does no harm, to a very dangerous situation for both mother and baby.

If you have a placental abruption, you will usually see some bleeding and feel abdominal pain. The baby may be in distress as well. Separation at the edge of the placenta causes the most bleeding, but because it is not near the umbilical cord, it may be less risky to the fetus. If the central part of the placenta separates, there may be hardly any vaginal bleeding, but the fetus is at great risk. In other words, you can't judge how serious this is by the amount of bleeding you experience.

Often an ultrasound can identify an abruption, but sometimes it is hard to recognize. Significant abruptions usually make labor start. Big abruptions, as well as threatening the life of the fetus, can cause abnormalities in the clotting of the mother's blood.

Treatment of abruption depends completely on its severity. If it is minor, the bleeding may stop on its own, the baby will be fine and the pregnancy can continue to term. If it is severe, though, the mother may need intravenous fluids and blood transfusions to treat her shock and clotting problems, and delivery of the baby is urgent. Each woman with a severe abruption must be assessed individually to decide if vaginal delivery or Caesarean section is a better choice.

Placenta Previa

A placenta previa is a placenta that is either partially or completely covering the cervix. This occurs in about 1 out of 200 births, and can be diagnosed by ultrasound.

Placenta previa causes painless vaginal bleeding, almost always before the onset of labor (only 2 percent of women with this condition have no bleeding until labor starts). If labor proceeds, this is a very dangerous situation because as the cervix opens, the placenta will bleed very heavily. Caesarean section is the treatment, and is life-saving for the mother.

The risk to the baby depends on how premature it is when the Caesarean section has to be performed because of bleeding. If the baby is at term, both mother and baby should do well.

A pelvic examination should never be performed when placenta previa is suspected, as even touching the cervix when the placenta is implanted over it can start heavy bleeding.

> ### The Evidence About...
> ### MISCARRIAGE
>
> **Miscarriage is a common pregnancy complication that cannot be prevented. Women who miscarry need emotional support as well as physical care.**
>
> **The tragedy of DES should remind all of us about the importance of research. The research showed that DES did not prevent miscarriage, yet many doctors continued using it. As well, this hormone was assumed to be safe because babies appeared normal at birth; it was only years later that researchers discovered its tragic, long-term effects.**

been normal. How could she say that? I wanted that baby so much. She just made me feel awful, like I couldn't have a normal baby. I needed her to at least say she was sorry, not to tell me to be grateful."

Charlene felt she coped quite well after experiencing an early miscarriage, but when her "due date" arrived, she felt sad all day long. "I couldn't get it out of my mind that this was the day my baby was supposed to be born," she says.

Women may benefit at some time from information about miscarriage, most particularly from the knowledge that it is common, and that nothing they did caused it or could

have prevented it. But they also need an acknowledgement of their grief: that this has been a loss they can mourn.

Fathers, too, can be deeply affected by a miscarriage. Early on, the pregnancy may not seem entirely real to some fathers, but dads also join in the planning and the excitement and feel the loss when a pregnancy ends unexpectedly.

"It was seeing the ultrasound that did it for me," says Rod. "I was so impressed when I could see his little heart beating. I knew he was real, I knew he was alive. And then we lost him. I think I felt as bad as Janine, even though I didn't have to go through the physical stuff."

Julie had two miscarriages and then gave birth to a healthy, full-term baby. "I was just devastated when I had the second miscarriage. The first time I made out that it was no big deal, miscarriages are pretty common. But when it happened again, I began to feel like I would never have a baby. When I told my doctor how miserable I was feeling—I'd go to work and end up crying in the washroom—she referred me to a support group and that helped a lot."

Support groups such as the one Julie joined are available in many communities; other women have found comfort through making connections in newsletters, books and through the Internet with other women who have had miscarriages. Ask your physician or midwife about what is available in your area, if you would like some extra support.

15

How Is Your Baby Lying? Unusual Presentations

Your doctor presses her hands against your very pregnant belly, slides them down towards your pelvis and announces, "Feels like a vertex presentation, probably anterior."

It might sound like a foreign language, but all your doctor means is that your baby is in the most common position: head down, with its face towards your backbone. The word "presentation" means the baby's position inside the uterus; the part of the baby's body that comes out of your vagina first is called the "presenting part."

About 95 percent of babies are head-down at the time of birth—this is called a cephalic, or a vertex, presentation. Earlier in pregnancy, when the baby is smaller, its position will change frequently as it moves around inside the uterus. The baby will be head-down sometimes and feet-down at other times. Probably because the baby's head is normally the heaviest

This is the most common presentation. The baby is head-down (vertex) and, although angled a little to one side, the back of the head is down the mother's front.

In the posterior position, the baby is again head-down and slightly to one side, but the back of the head is towards the mother's spine. The increased pressure against the spine frequently causes backache during labor.

part of its body, it will usually settle into a head-down position a few weeks before birth.

Even with head-first babies, though, there are some variations.

Posterior Position

About one in four babies will be in a *posterior* position during labor. This means that the baby is head-down but its face is towards the mother's stomach. Often the baby will rotate around to the more common *anterior* position (with the face towards the mother's back)

either during labor or at the time of birth, but as long as the baby is in the posterior position, labor is likely to be longer and more painful.

Susan's third child was posterior, and the intense back pain she felt during this labor took her by surprise. "With Zoe, my posterior baby, when the contractions went away, the pain didn't stop. It wasn't as intense as when I was having a contraction, but it was a strong ache in my back. And the labor went on and on—18 hours altogether."

Susan found that having steady pressure on her back right at the center of the pain was most helpful. She also spent a good part of her labor kneeling on the bed. "I walked around with the other two, but walking made me feel worse with Zoe. So I knelt on the bed and rocked."

After 18 hours, Susan says, "I felt something move. I didn't know what it was, but I yelled to Steve—who was still patiently rubbing my back—to call the nurse. Zoe had finally turned, and she was born within a couple of minutes. The doctor just barely made it."

Most babies in a posterior position, like Zoe, will turn spontaneously at some time during the labor and be born in the usual position, with their faces looking down. Some babies will stay in a posterior position and will be born face-up. This is unusual and usually causes some comment in the delivery room—these babies are referred to as being "sunny-side up."

When a baby stays in the posterior position, it is more difficult to push out, and some women will push for a long period of time without making much progress. In these cases, the doctor will usually suggest helping to get the baby out with a vacuum extractor or forceps. The mother will usually be given an epidural, and then the doctor will either try to turn the baby into an anterior position so that it can be pushed out more easily, or will deliver the baby in the posterior position.

A Face-First Baby

Elizabeth was in hard labor with her second baby. "How much longer do you think it will be?" she asked her doctor.

The doctor did a pelvic exam and looked puzzled. "Well, Elizabeth, I'm not feeling what I'm expecting to find," she said. "The cervix is well over half dilated, but the presenting part of the baby doesn't feel like a head; it feels soft."

"Does that mean something's wrong with the baby?" Elizabeth asked in a panic. Suddenly the pain of the contractions felt like nothing compared to this new worry.

"I don't know. I just can't tell what I'm feeling. I'll get the radiologist to come and do an ultrasound. That should tell us what's what."

The radiologist, called out of bed at 3:00 a.m., showed up 10 minutes later in shorts and sandals. He could see how worried Elizabeth and her doctor were, and the ultrasound was quickly arranged. It showed that the baby was in a face presentation.

"The soft, squishy things I was feeling are the baby's lips and cheeks—I'm glad I was gentle!" laughed the doctor.

"But can I get the baby out in this position? I almost feel like I have to push already," asked Elizabeth.

She had had an easy labor with her first baby, who was over eight pounds. The doctor was obviously not worried, now that she knew what she had been feeling in the vagina. "Your labor seems to be going fast. I'm sure you'll be able to deliver this baby. But be prepared for the face to look really swollen and bruised."

Elizabeth says, "The actual birth was amazing. The pushing felt just like with my first baby, but it went a lot faster. After just a couple of big pushes, I could feel the burning at the opening. The doctor had set a mirror up so I could watch. The first thing we saw were these swollen purple things. As the baby came further out, we realized they were his lips! Then came the cheeks, then the whole rest of the head and body. He started crying right away, so I knew he was fine, but did he ever look funny. His lips and cheeks were so swollen, his face looked like a little piggy. That disappeared within a few days, and he was as handsome as his dad."

Sometimes it becomes clear that the posterior baby is not going to turn, and is not going to fit through the mother's pelvis in this position. Then a Caesarean section may be the safest course for both mother and baby. Each situation must be evaluated individually.

Face or Brow Presentation

In less than 1 percent of pregnancies, the baby will be head-down but have its neck arched, so that either its face or forehead is coming through the vagina first. Usually, the labor contractions will gradually change this position to the more common chin-tucked-in position. If the baby remains with the forehead first (called a brow presentation), a Caesarean section is usually necessary, as this presentation of the baby's head does not fit through the birth canal. If the baby's neck really arches so that the face actually presents, the baby can often be born vaginally.

Compound Presentation

Lesley's first child was a compound presentation. She says, "My water broke several days

A frank breech presentation, with the baby's legs folded up against his body. Some breech babies "sit" in the pelvis with their legs crossed (complete breech), or even extend one or both legs straight down (footling breech).

after Melissa was due, and I went into labor right away. Labor was pretty intense, but short, and I didn't need much medication. But the pushing stage was really hard and long and more painful than I had expected."

The reason for that unexpectedly difficult pushing stage was clear as soon as baby Melissa emerged. Her left arm was extended beside her head; the pressure of the birth left an imprint of her hand on the side of her face that lasted for several days.

A compound presentation means that more than one part of the baby is trying to get through the birth canal at once. In some cases, like Lesley's, it merely makes the birth more difficult; in other cases, vaginal birth is impossible and a Caesarean section is necessary. Compound presentation cannot be diagnosed before labor, as babies move around in the uterus, and even during labor the baby's position can shift.

Breech Presentation

Some babies take a completely opposite approach to birth—they want to come bottom- or feet-first. This is known as a *breech* presentation. About 15 percent of babies are breech at 29 to 32 weeks, and between 3 and 4 percent will still be breech when labor begins. Once labor is active, it is unlikely that the baby will turn by itself because of the tightness of the uterus—however, some do "flip over" during labor.

Turning Breech Babies

Linda, whose son Joshua is now two years old, was told by her midwife that Joshua was in a breech position when she was 32 weeks pregnant. The midwife suggested she try some positioning exercises—"basically having my bum stuck up in the air"—two or three times a day to see if the baby would turn head-down, but it didn't work. She also visited another midwife who attempted an "external version." This is a technique to turn the baby into a head-down position by manipulating the baby through the mother's abdomen. This was also unsuccessful.

At 37 weeks, Linda went to an obstetrician and a second attempt at external version was made. She had an intravenous started and was given ritodrine, a drug to relax her uterus. Linda had both the obstetrician and an intern working together to move her baby and "it felt like the baby was going to come out of my mouth while they were doing it." Twenty minutes later, her baby was head-down, and three weeks later Joshua was born vaginally. "Yes," she says, "it was well worth the trouble we went to to get him turned around."

Strategies to turn a breech baby into the more favorable head-down position include exercises for the mother—such as the ones Linda tried—and a technique called "external version" of the baby.

EXERCISES

Midwives have often suggested "exercises" for women to do to turn breech babies. In one, the mother lies on her back, flexes her hips and knees and rolls from side to side for five or ten minutes. In another, the mother kneels on her hands and knees on the floor and someone else shakes the uterus for a few minutes.

In the third exercise, the only one to have been studied at all, the mother kneels on the floor with her hips flexed a bit but not pressing on her abdomen, and her head and shoulders on the floor, for 15 minutes three times a day. The single uncontrolled study of this method found no difference in outcome that could not have been caused by chance.

EXTERNAL VERSION

External version, when done by a doctor, is usually performed in hospital. Usually a recording of the baby's heart rate is done first for 15 or 20 minutes. An ultrasound is used to locate the placenta and the umbilical cord and to identify the exact position of the baby's legs. The physician puts his hands on the mother's abdomen and tries to rotate the baby, watching the ultrasound to make sure that the heart rate remains normal.

Some breech positions will turn more easily than others. If the baby has its hips and knees bent so it is all curled up, the version is most likely to succeed. If the baby's legs are sticking straight up, or if they are dangling down into the pelvis, version is less likely to work.

External version has some risks. It is safest if it is performed with continuous ultrasound, so that the position of the placenta can be seen and the fetal heart rate can be continuously monitored. Moving the baby can occasionally cause the placenta to be separated from the wall of the uterus, resulting in bleeding and fetal distress. (Rh negative mothers who are having versions should be given Rh immune globulin—see Chapter 17, Rh Negative Mother.) Being turned can also cause slowing of the baby's heart rate, presumably because of tangling or compression of the umbilical cord. If fetal distress occurs, the doctor will stop trying to turn the baby, and if the heart rate does not improve promptly, a Caesarean section may be needed.

Lisa was about 34 weeks pregnant with her second child when the doctor told her the baby was in a breech position. "I knew something was different from my first pregnancy. I could feel a hard bump under my ribs that wasn't there when I was pregnant with Olivia."

Her doctor scheduled an ultrasound when Lisa was 37 weeks pregnant and the baby's position hadn't changed. "I have to admit I was scared. My doctor offered us the option of trying a version. We went into the hospital, and the doctor explained that if the version caused fetal distress, he would need to do an immediate Caesarean section. I also knew that it could bring on labor, so I had Gary and my labor support person with me as well."

Lisa was settled in bed and attached to an ultrasound machine and a fetal monitor. "The baby's heart rate was great, and we could all see her little head right up under my ribs." After a few minutes, to be sure the heart rate was stable, the obstetrician placed his hand behind the bump on Lisa's stomach that showed where her baby's head was, and pushed. "It was a bit uncomfortable but not as bad as I had thought it might be. And it was over much faster than I had expected."

Watching the ultrasound while he maneuvered the baby into position, Lisa's doctor made sure that the baby wasn't tangled in the umbilical cord or showing signs of distress. Within a few minutes, her baby was head-down. Lisa stayed sitting up in her hospital bed for another hour while nurses monitored the baby's heart rate, but the actual procedure had taken only five minutes. That evening she walked around a lot, hoping it would help the baby's head settle deeper into her pelvis.

"I worried that the baby would flip back, but she didn't," Lisa says. And five weeks later, she delivered a nine-pound baby girl—head-first—after a short, straightforward labor.

WHEN SHOULD YOU TRY EXTERNAL VERSION?

Turning the breech baby before 37 weeks is fairly easy, as the baby is small and there is a large amount of amniotic fluid. However, the baby so often just flips back to the breech position again that it does not prevent breech presentations at the time of delivery.

Waiting until 37 weeks or after is a better choice. The baby may flip into a head-down position on its own by that time. It also allows enough time for complications like placenta previa—which will require a Caesarean delivery anyway—to show up. At 37 weeks the baby is mature enough to be born, so if the version does cause a separation of the placenta or fetal distress from tangling the cord, the baby can be delivered promptly by Caesarean section without running the risks of prematurity.

External version after 37 weeks reduces the chance of the baby being breech at delivery.

EXTERNAL VERSION IN EARLY LABOR

Turning of breech in early labor has been reported to be successful in 75 percent of cases, but the studies have been very small. Using drugs to relax the uterus may increase the success rate of the procedure and reduce the amount of force needed.

Complications of Vaginal Breech Delivery

The reason that so much attention has been paid to turning breech babies into a head-down position is that a breech birth is associated with a higher rate of injury and death for the baby. (Breech babies do tend to have a higher rate of congenital abnormalities, so not all of the risk is due to the delivery itself.)

The delivery of a breech baby is more difficult than for a head-down baby. Because the relatively small and soft buttocks and legs deliver first, the perineum does not get very stretched. Then the larger head and shoulders have to maneuver through the vagina quickly so the baby can start breathing. For this reason, episiotomy in a breech delivery is often done to speed up the birth.

If the baby is coming feet-first rather than buttocks-first, there is a 15 percent risk of "cord prolapse"—the umbilical cord slipping through the cervix ahead of the baby. This is dangerous because the cord will be compressed and cut off the baby's oxygen supply. An emergency Caesarean section is the treatment.

Breech birth is riskier for premature babies, because their tiny legs and buttocks may deliver before the cervix is fully dilated; then the relatively large head may be trapped. This can lead to a very difficult delivery with possible injury to the baby's head.

Caesarean Section versus Breech Vaginal Delivery

Some physicians recommend Caesarean section for all breech babies without even waiting for labor to start. Many physicians recommend

Caesarean section if it is a first baby, if the baby is estimated to be over eight pounds, or if it is a footling breech (the feet coming before the buttocks). Their concern is that during a vaginal delivery the baby's body will be delivered and then the head, coming last, will prove to be too large for the mother's pelvis and be stuck.

There is very little research to support (or refute) these recommendations. The only studies that have been done to compare Caesarean section with vaginal birth for babies in a breech position have been very small. In the Caesarean section group, they found a small decrease in short-term complications for the baby, but an increase in complications for the mother. The numbers, however, were too small to be meaningful.

At present, advice is given solely on the individual preference of the obstetrician involved. In the summer of 1997, plans were announced for an international study of 2800 women at 75 hospitals to compare vaginal and Caesarean delivery of breech babies. The study leader, Dr. Mary Hannah of the University of Toronto, explained: "We need solid evidence that doctors can use to help their patients make the best decision about their birth. We don't really know the benefits of these two approaches, vaginal delivery or Caesarean section for breech. We feel some urgency. Younger obstetricians in training programs aren't getting a lot of experience in delivering a breech birth vaginally. It's easier for them to do a Caesarean because they're more experienced at that. We felt if we didn't resolve the issue soon, vaginal delivery would no longer be an option to women with a breech."

This is a well-designed, randomized trial that should answer the question being asked. There are two potential problems that may come up. Will a large enough number of women consent to enter the trial and be randomly assigned to vaginal delivery or Caesarean section? Will the physicians doing the vaginal deliveries have the experience and confidence to manage the vaginal breech births, or will they tend to switch over to a Caesarean delivery—which, as Dr. Hannah says, is easier for the doctor? Time will tell.

Transverse Lie

Approximately 1 in 500 babies will be in a "transverse" position—lying at right angles to the birth canal with perhaps a shoulder or arm as the presenting part. (This is

A transverse lie. If the baby can't be turned by external version, a Caesarean delivery will be required.

completely different from the *head* being in a transverse position in the birth canal, which means that it is rotated halfway between anterior and posterior.)

About 80 percent of babies in a transverse lie at 37 weeks will move to a normal head-down position before delivery, so usually the physician or midwife will simply wait and see.

In early labor, if the baby is still in a transverse position, it is worth trying external version—pushing the baby into a head-down position by manipulating through the mother's belly. The success rate for this isn't very high, but if the baby doesn't move, a Caesarean section will be needed.

The Evidence About...
HOW YOUR BABY IS LYING

Labor is the best test of how the baby will fit through the pelvis; no estimates made before labor are very useful.

Using external version to turn breech babies after 37 weeks substantially reduces the chance of the baby being breech in labor. This reduces the risk of Caesarean section.

The safest method of delivery for breech babies, whether vaginal or Caesarean section, has not been established.

16

More than One Baby: Multiple Pregnancy

When Diane's first son Craig was 10 months old, she and her husband decided to try for another baby. She conceived almost immediately, and early in the pregnancy her doctor noticed how big she was getting and recommended an ultrasound. The ultrasound, Diane says, "began an adventure that still seems quite incredible" when it showed that she was carrying four (yes, four) babies.

Although she had not been sick at all during her first pregnancy, Diane experienced severe nausea and vomiting the second time. Her mother came to stay with the family and to help care for Diane's toddler over the next few stressful months.

Diane was admitted to hospital at 24 weeks gestation because she was having occasional contractions. "I was told I'd have a Caesarean for the delivery because there were just too many things that could get tangled up, but the doctors waited until I went into labor." Her quadruplets, two boys (Harrison and Kenny) and two girls (Alison and Jessica), were born at 27 weeks gestation. They weighed 2 lbs. 5 ½ oz., 2 lbs. 6 oz., 2 lbs. 8 oz. and 3 lbs. ½ oz.

"All four of them needed respirators," Diane says, "and before they were born the nurses would say to me that I couldn't go into labor today because there were only three respirators available. Fortunately, I went into labor on a four-respirator day."

The quadruplets stayed in the hospital for two and a half months, and, as Diane says, "experienced practically every problem you can think of that a premature baby could have." But all four arrived home healthy and have continued to do very well.

Diane says people meeting their family often say, "I'm glad it's you and not me." When she hears those words she thinks to herself, "I'm glad it's me, too." She tells other parents expecting multiples: "Yes, it's hard, it's not what you had planned, but it's also very joyous and very special."

Diane's story is a dramatic and uncommon one. Quadruplets are very rare, although they (and other multiple births, from twins and

Fertility Treatments and Multiple Births

When women are having trouble conceiving, they may be given medications to encourage ovulation–but this medication often causes more than one egg to be released during each menstrual cycle. This increases the chances of having at least one egg fertilized, but if several eggs are fertilized, the women will become pregnant with twins, triplets or more babies.

Another approach to treating infertility involves removing eggs from the mother's ovaries during surgery, fertilizing the eggs with sperm outside her body and then implanting these fertilized eggs in her uterus. Because many of these implanted eggs will not survive, usually several are implanted at the same time. If two or more do survive, though, the mother will find herself with a multiple pregnancy.

The increased use of these treatments is the main reason we are seeing multiple births more frequently.

triplets to septuplets) are becoming more common with the increasing use of fertility drugs. (Diane, however, did not use any fertility drugs.) The most common multiple pregnancy, of course, produces twins.

Twins are born about 1 out of every 90 births in North America. Identical twins arise from a single fertilized egg that divides in the first few days after conception. The number of identical twins is about 1 out of every 250 births; this is remarkably constant worldwide and seems unrelated to age, heredity, number of other children or race. Identical twins are truly "chance" occurrences.

Fraternal twins arise from the separate fertilization of two eggs, both of which are released in the same menstrual cycle. The frequency of fraternal twins varies considerably. In rural Nigeria, twinning occurs once in 20 births. In Japan, twinning occurs only once in 155 births. Heredity is important—a mother who is a twin is much more likely to have twins. Fraternal twinning is more common the older the mother is and the more children she has had. Fraternal twinning is more common in big, tall women. And yes, fraternal twins can have two different fathers.

The number of twin pregnancies is far higher than the number of twin births. The introduction of very early ultrasound has shown that many twin pregnancies end early on with the spontaneous death and reabsorption of one twin. Probably, some cases of "threatened miscarriage" actually are the miscarriage of a twin while the other twin survives and goes on to a full-term delivery. There have been rare cases of twins delivering at different times, occasionally weeks apart, but almost always both babies were very premature.

A multiple birth—twins, triplets or even more—is both exciting and stressful. A woman carrying more than one baby is likely to experience common pregnancy symptoms (heartburn, nausea, fatigue, etc.) more severely than a woman carrying a single child. She may also feel anxious about the emotional and financial aspects of taking care of more than one infant.

Multiple pregnancies are at a higher risk for a number of pregnancy problems. If you are expecting twins, triplets or more, you are much more likely to go into labor prematurely. You are more likely to develop pre-eclampsia. Your babies are more likely to be small for gestational age, as well as premature. The combination of prematurity and being small for gestational age makes the risk of perinatal death and cerebral palsy higher than in single births.

If you discover that you are expecting more than one baby, you may find a support group extremely helpful. Knowing other parents who have survived (and enjoyed) the experience of caring for more than one newborn will be reassuring, and these parents will probably have plenty of tips on getting through the pregnancy as well.

Treatment Options

For many years, bed rest has been recommended for women with a multiple pregnancy. The goal is to help the babies grow bigger and to reduce premature labor. Bed rest, either in or out of hospital, was introduced into clinical practice before its risks or benefits were ever evaluated by research.

Very little research has been conducted on bed rest, and most of it deals with twins rather than pregnancies with more than two babies. The research has not produced clear or consistent results.

Some studies have shown that hospitalization reduces the rate of high blood pressure in mothers, but causes no improvement in any other outcome.

A study involving women who had shown some early dilation of the cervix (which would suggest they were more likely to go into labor prematurely) did not show any differences in the rate of premature birth between the "bed rest in hospital" group and the control group.

The research also suggests that the number of babies born prematurely, as well as

the number with a very low birth weight, is actually higher when mothers are routinely hospitalized.

Bed rest seems like an impossible goal for some. Maureen had two-year-old twins when she became pregnant again—with twins. "I was advised to rest as much as possible," she says, "but how much rest can you get with a couple of two-year-olds to look after? It didn't seem to make a lot of difference. I went into labor at 37 weeks—just like the first time—and the babies were both a good size and healthy."

Various medications to prevent premature labor in multiple pregnancies have also been tested, and none have been shown to be effective.

How should your twins or other multiples be born—vaginally or by Caesarean section? Again, this has not been well researched, although there is more information about twins than other multiple births. One study compared Caesarean section to vaginal birth when the second twin was breech. The researchers found that the mothers who had Caesarean sections were more likely to have complications, and there were no benefits in terms of the outcomes for the babies. Triplets and higher multiples are almost always delivered by Caesarean section, but this is not on the basis of any research evidence.

Because multiple births—especially those involving more than two babies—are less common than single pregnancies, it is harder to conduct research on them, and there are no definitive answers to many questions. This means that parents expecting multiples, and the caregivers who are working with them, have less concrete information on which to base decisions.

The Evidence About . . .
TWINS AND HIGHER MULTIPLES

Additional advice and support is helpful for parents who find they are having more than one baby.

No evidence supports the widely given advice to women pregnant with twins to rest more, or to be admitted to hospital to rest.

Research does not support the routine use of Caesarean section for all twin births.

Research on the best care for higher multiple births is minimal, due in part to the difficulty in studying a relatively rare occurrence. However, the increased use of fertility drugs means that these multiple births are becoming more common.

17

Rh Negative Mother

At your last prenatal appointment, a sample of your blood was taken to test your blood type. Today, when you sit down beside your doctor's desk, she says, "I see that you're Rh negative. We should talk about giving you the Rh gammaglobulin. Do you know the blood type of the baby's father?"

"No," you say, puzzled. "I can ask him. But why does it matter?"

Your doctor explains: "If he is Rh negative like you, we don't need to worry, because your baby has to be Rh negative as well. If he is Rh positive, then your baby might be Rh positive, and there may be a problem in that situation."

What does it mean to be Rh negative, and how will this affect your baby?

You might have heard about babies who died in the past because their mothers were Rh negative when the baby was Rh positive. Today the problem is rare; a drug called anti-D gammaglobulin can prevent almost all Rh problems.

If you have ever donated blood, you will have a card listing your blood type. In one cat-egory, you can be A, B, AB or O. In another category, you can be Rh positive (this means you have a substance called factor D in your blood) or Rh negative (you don't have factor D). Your card will describe your blood type as, for example, A negative or O positive.

About 15 percent of white North Americans are Rh negative; among black North Americans, only 7 to 8 percent are Rh negative.

If the mother is Rh positive and the baby is Rh negative, there is no problem. If the mother and the baby are both Rh negative or both Rh positive, that does not cause a problem, either. The *only* time there may be a problem is if the mother is Rh negative and the baby is Rh positive.

When Jennifer found out that she was Rh negative, she asked her husband what his blood type was. He turned out to be Rh negative as well. "Great," Jennifer's doctor told her. "You two are obviously a good match! We don't need to worry about the gammaglobulin in this situation."

But Trudy's case was different. Her husband

Hemolytic Disease of the Newborn

In the days before anti-D gammaglobulin, not all Rh negative women had problems. In fact, the majority did not. Only about 17 percent of Rh negative women develop antibodies, and only some of their babies become ill. However, this is still a substantial number, and the disease can be very serious.

While the antibodies in her blood will cause no symptoms in the mother, they can cross the placenta during her next pregnancy, get into her baby's blood system and break down (hemolyze) its red cells.

In the most severe cases, the baby dies in the uterus. In less severe cases, the fetus becomes very anemic. This can be discovered by amniocentesis, and is treated with blood transfusions. If the baby is too premature to be born, it can be given transfusions inside the uterus. As soon as the baby is mature enough, labor is induced so the baby can be transfused outside the uterus.

Babies born with severe hemolytic disease often need immediate resuscitation and blood transfusions. Less severely affected babies are well at birth, but quickly develop jaundice (yellowness of the skin) as bilirubin accumulates in their blood. Bilirubin is produced when red blood cells are broken down. To prevent brain damage from high levels of bilirubin, jaundice *above a certain level* is treated with special fluorescent lights that reduce the level of bilirubin in the blood. (Mild jaundice is common and normal in newborns, and does not usually require treatment.) If this phototherapy is not sufficient, blood transfusion is required.

tested Rh positive, and the doctor explained that there might be a problem. "Your baby could inherit the Rh positive blood type from Eric," the doctor pointed out, "and then there is a risk of you developing antibodies against the Rh positive blood cells."

The problem with the Rh negative mother and her Rh positive baby develops when blood from the baby mixes with the mother's blood. The mother's and fetus' blood circulations are in completely separate blood vessels, but these vessels are very close to one another in the placenta. Little ruptures can occur in the placenta, and blood cells from the baby can enter the mother's circulation.

When the baby's Rh positive blood cells get into the mother's Rh negative circulation, the mother's immune system will recognize them as foreign and make antibodies against them: these are called anti-D antibodies. Like the antibodies we make to kill germs, anti-D antibodies attack cells—in this case, Rh positive red blood cells.

The time when this mingling of blood cells is most likely to happen is right after delivery, when the placenta is separating from the wall of the uterus. The baby is already born, so even if these antibodies do form, the baby can't be harmed by them.

There is almost no risk to the first baby, even if it is Rh positive and the mother is Rh negative. But these antibodies stay in the mother's circulation, so if she gets pregnant again with another Rh positive baby, they can easily cross the placenta and attack that baby's red blood cells, causing a disease called *hemolytic disease of the newborn*.

This problem was more serious in the past, when women tended to have larger families: with each baby, the risks increased. The smaller families that are common today, and the availability of effective preventive treatment, mean that Rh incompatibility problems are far less likely.

Preventing Anti-D Antibodies from Forming

Anti-D gammaglobulin is a concentrated, purified blood product that is given to the Rh negative mother. It coats any Rh positive cells entering her circulation and keeps them from causing the production of antibodies.

When the Rh negative mother gives birth, a sample of the baby's blood is taken from the umbilical cord and tested. If the baby is Rh negative, there is no problem and nothing needs to be done.

If the baby is Rh positive, an injection of anti-D gammaglobulin is given to the mother. This should be given within 72 hours of delivery. Before the development of anti-D gammaglobulin, about 17 percent of Rh negative women who delivered an Rh positive baby would show anti-D antibodies in their blood at the beginning of their next pregnancy. *With the use of anti-D gammaglobulin, the risk of antibodies in the next pregnancy is reduced from 17 percent to 0.2 percent.*

There are other times when the mother's and baby's blood can mix. Anti-D gammaglobulin given at these other times reduces still further the chance of antibody production. These risky situations are discussed below.

After a Miscarriage or Induced Abortion

If given after an abortion or miscarriage to all Rh negative mothers, anti-D gammaglobulin reduces the risk of sensitization from around 3 percent to 0.2 percent. Obviously, this method treats all the women who had Rh negative fetuses as well, but since the blood type of the fetus is unobtainable, the safest course is to treat everyone.

"I couldn't understand why my doctor wanted me to have this shot after my miscarriage," Eleanor says. "It seemed like one more thing to cope with when I was feeling so miserable about losing the baby." But when she thought it over, she decided to take the gammaglobulin. "It got me thinking about my next baby and doing what I could to protect him or her," Eleanor recalls. "In a funny way, it gave me some hope."

After Bleeding during the Pregnancy

Anti-D gammaglobulin is recommended after any procedure that might cause bleeding from the placenta during pregnancy. These include amniocentesis, chorionic villus biopsy, significant abdominal injury to the mother, abruption of the placenta or external version of a breech baby.

Because the blood type of the fetus is not known during the pregnancy, this also treats some mothers with Rh negative fetuses. The gammaglobulin is not dangerous or harmful to the baby whether it is Rh negative or Rh positive.

Treating All Rh Negative Mothers Routinely during Pregnancy

A small number of Rh negative women carrying an Rh positive baby will develop Rh antibodies during their first pregnancy, even before they deliver. Some researchers have tried giving all Rh negative women anti-D gammaglobulin at 28 weeks of pregnancy. The blood type of the baby was checked at birth, and those mothers who had an Rh positive baby were given a second injection of anti-D gammaglobulin within 72 hours of birth. Adding this 28-week injection further reduced the risk of sensitization from 0.2 percent to 0.06 percent.

Is Anti-D Gammaglobulin Safe?

Anti-D gammaglobulin is a blood product and must be screened for hepatitis and HIV, as other blood products are. The method of extraction of the gammaglobulin kills the HIV virus. Women who have religious objections to blood products must make their own decisions about its use. Otherwise, there are no known complications from this treatment.

The Evidence About...
Rh NEGATIVE MOTHERS

With the use of anti-D gammaglobulin, the risk of antibody production in Rh negative women can be reduced to 0.06 percent.

All women should have their blood tested in early pregnancy to see if they are Rh negative and if they have anti-D antibodies.

For Rh negative women without antibodies, treatment with anti-D gammaglobulin after a miscarriage or after delivery of an Rh positive baby can prevent antibody formation and dramatically reduce the risk of hemolytic disease of the newborn in another pregnancy.

In situations where the fetal blood and maternal blood may mix, such as amniocentesis or a placental abruption, anti-D gammaglobulin given as soon as possible can significantly reduce the risk to this baby and subsequent babies.

Routine treatment of all Rh negative pregnancies at 28 weeks does give a small further benefit.

Women who already have antibodies (fortunately rare since the introduction of gammaglobulin) need to have their pregnancies carefully followed in a specialized center where the baby's need for intra-uterine transfusion, premature delivery or transfusion after birth can be assessed.

Part Four

Giving Birth to Your Baby

Riziero Vertolli

After nine months of waiting and wondering what it will be like, the day of your baby's birth has finally arrived. Every birth is unique, but many of the concerns and questions expectant mothers have are universal. How much will it hurt? How will I cope with the pain? How long will it take? Will my baby be okay?

The day your baby is born will be a day you will never forget. You can't really plan or predict what will happen, but you can take some steps to make the experience as positive as possible.

Here's the best evidence about giving birth, on everything from figuring out when you're in labor and avoiding unhelpful hospital routines to pushing your baby out.

18

Arriving at the Hospital: Hospital Routines and Labor Support

"Okay, honey, we're here." Your husband scoots around the car and opens the door and you climb out awkwardly. (It's at least nice to think that the next time you get out of the car your big belly won't be in the way.) Before you can walk into the hospital, another contraction hits and you lean on your husband as he gently rubs your back.

As the hospital doors slide open, you walk through. What happens next will depend a great deal on which hospital you have chosen to give birth in. Each hospital has its own policies and routines, and the variations can be quite dramatic even within the same geographic area.

What are some of the routines you may encounter—and what steps can you take if you want to avoid them? Always remember that just because something is routine at your particular hospital, that doesn't make it mandatory.

In most hospitals, you will have to stop at the admitting department and register before going to labor and delivery. Some hospitals arrange for you to send in pre-registration forms ahead of time (or you can arrange this for yourself by checking with your hospital), but there is still a stop at the admitting department to let them know you have arrived and to pick up forms to take to labor and delivery. Sometimes the mother can go straight to labor and delivery and her partner can take care of the admission routines (be sure he has your birth date, insurance information, etc.!).

When you arrive at labor and delivery, the nurse will start to make out your chart. She will want to hear about when the contractions started and how close together they are. She'll ask if there has been any bloody show or if the membranes have ruptured yet. She'll also ask some questions about your past health, your previous pregnancies and how this pregnancy has gone, particularly about any special tests you may have had. All this will be written down on your chart.

Then the nurse will take your blood pressure, your temperature and your pulse, and ask you to pee into a bottle. She may do a vaginal examination as well. If you are in a teaching hospital, the intern or resident may come to see you, may ask some of the same questions the nurse just asked and may be the one to do the vaginal exam rather than the nurse.

Sometimes your partner and/or support people will be asked to leave during this initial examination; you can ask that they stay with you. You will be offered a hospital gown to wear but you can bring a comfortable nightgown from home instead, if you prefer. A bathrobe can also be useful, so that you won't feel as exposed as you walk around.

None of this admission procedure will be much of a problem if you are in early labor. If you've come in during very hard labor, responding to the nurse will be more difficult, and can break the concentration you are using to deal with your contractions. From the hospital's point of view, the paperwork is very important and has to be done.

Many hospitals ask all mothers to have the electronic fetal monitor attached for 20 minutes after admission, to provide a paper printout of the baby's heart rate to assess the baby's condition. The theory is that babies who need more intensive monitoring can be identified during this period of time. This has not been researched, so we do not know if it has any value. You are entitled to decide not to have the 20-minute strip done—just say you don't want to do it.

Patricia says, "When I arrived at the hospital in labor, the nurse said I had to have a 20-minute strip done. Well, I guess she was busy because she didn't come back to take me off the machine for over an hour. I was really uncomfortable lying there, my back hurt so much. But that wasn't the worst part. The worst was that Jeff was paying more attention to the machine than to me. He'd watch the

Hospital Routines to Avoid

Research shows that some kinds of care women in labor may receive are *not* beneficial when used routinely (although some of these can be useful in specific situations).

During labor:

- routine enema;
- routine shaving of pubic hair;
- routine continuous electronic fetal monitoring;
- rectal examinations (rather than vaginal) to check the cervix;
- routinely withholding food and drink;
- routine use of IV fluids;
- regularly scheduled vaginal examinations;
- keeping women in bed;
- having a 20-minute session of continuous electronic fetal monitoring.

During the pushing stage and birth:

- having the woman lying on her back with her legs up in stirrups to push the baby out;
- routine or liberal use of episiotomy;
- routine directed pushing;
- pushing with the mother holding her breath and sustained bearing down;
- encouraging bearing down or pushing as soon as the cervix is fully dilated;
- routine use of vacuum extractor or forceps to shorten the pushing stage.

graph and tell me when a contraction was coming—as if I couldn't feel it myself. Then he'd stare at the numbers, while I was trying to cope with the pain. I was so glad when she finally took it off and we could get up and walk around. Next time, I'm going to refuse to have it put on at all."

Enemas to empty the bowels were, at one time, given to most laboring women when they arrived at the hospital. They are still routine at a few hospitals. However, two studies found that enemas did not shorten labor, that there were no benefits in terms of infection rates and that most of the women given enemas found them unpleasant and uncomfortable. During the pushing stage, many women do pass stool as the baby pushes past the opening of the bowel. This is easily cleaned up and not necessarily prevented by having an enema. If enemas are given routinely at your hospital, you can decline if you wish.

Another once-common routine that is still followed in a few hospitals is shaving of pubic hair. The goal was to reduce infection and make any stitching that was needed easier, even though women found it quite uncomfortable when the hair grew back. However, two studies found that the rate of infection was actually higher for women who had been shaved. Since it increases the rate of infection, this is another routine that you might be wise to refuse if it is still done at your hospital.

Should you eat and drink during labor? Hospitals frequently have restrictions on whether women can eat or drink. In one survey, none of the hospitals studied allowed women to eat and drink as they wanted. Most allowed ice chips or sips of clear fluids, but no solid foods at all.

Why are these restrictions in place? The concern is that if an emergency situation arises that requires a Caesarean section under a general anesthetic, the mother may vomit and inhale some of the food into her lungs while she is unconscious from the anesthetic. The hope is that restricting food and drink during labor will guarantee an empty stomach in the rare situation that emergency general anesthesia is needed.

However, not eating or drinking after admission to the hospital during labor does not guarantee an empty stomach, because labor slows down the digestion of food—so food that you ate four hours before you arrived at the hospital could still be sitting in your stomach. Even if the mother's stomach has no food in it, it is still possible for the stomach acid to be inhaled during general anesthesia, causing burns to the lining of the lungs. This is a rare but serious problem. Taking antacids before you have the general anesthetic will reduce the acidity, but not prevent all cases of aspiration pneumonia.

In hospitals where mothers are not allowed to eat or drink, the policy may recommend giving the mother fluids and sugar intravenously instead. However, large volumes of sugar and water intravenously can result in both low blood sugar and low blood sodium in the newborn baby.

Most women are not hungry during active labor. A reasonable approach might be to allow women to eat and drink as they choose during their whole labor. Most women will choose easy-to-digest, small meals and will stop eating as labor becomes more intense. Continuing to drink fluids during labor avoids dehydration, avoids the possible complications of intravenous fluids and contributes only minimally to the risk of aspiration pneumonia in the rare situation in which general anesthesia is needed.

Position during labor and for delivery is sometimes dictated by hospital routine: some hospitals still encourage laboring women to stay in bed during their labor, either as a general policy or because they frequently use electronic fetal monitors. Lying in bed on your back, even if the head of the bed is raised, is probably the worst position for labor. The pressure of the uterus on the blood vessels when you are lying on your back means that there is less blood flow to the uterus. Contractions are not as strong or as effective in this position. Several studies have found that the baby is more likely to show signs of distress (a slow or irregular heartbeat), and labor progresses more slowly, when mothers lie on their backs.

So what position is better? Women who stand, walk or sit upright have shorter labors, on average, than women who lie in bed. Walking seems to be especially helpful in encouraging effective contractions. Women who walk or stay upright are less likely to use pain-relieving drugs, including epidurals. One study also found that babies born to mothers who walked around during labor had fewer abnormal heart rate recordings and higher Apgar scores, but other studies found no differences.

The Society of Obstetricians and Gynaecologists of Canada recommends that women be allowed to walk freely at all times during labor, to use baths or showers as they like and to choose their own positions for giving birth.

Hilary was in labor for about 30 hours and says, "I walked almost the whole time. At first, we walked around the neighborhood. Then when we got to the hospital, my contractions slowed down. I put my bathrobe on over the hospital gown and we went walking again. We walked all around the hospital, outside in the courtyard, into the parking lot and down the sidewalk. Every now and then I'd go back to the labor and delivery ward so the nurse could listen to the baby's heart." Hilary tried sitting in the whirlpool, but her contractions slowed down. "I had to get out and start walking again, it was the only way to keep my labor moving," she says.

Some labor and delivery units discourage women from leaving the department once they are admitted. This may mean there is literally no place to walk. You may be able to negotiate this, or if labor is still in the early stages, you might prefer to go home and return when you are closer to giving birth.

Labor Support—Comfort and Encouragement

Almost all hospitals now permit the woman's partner to stay with her throughout labor and

Labor Support—Comfort Techniques

Things your partner or other support person can do to make labor easier for you:

- massage your face, arms and legs to help you relax;
- gently stroke your belly;
- rub your back firmly to ease back pain;
- support you in an upright position during contractions;
- remind you of relaxing breathing patterns by breathing with you;

- help you find comfortable positions;
- put cold, wet cloths on your face, if you feel warm;
- give you ice, water or juice to drink;
- help you to develop a contraction "ritual" of breathing, humming, moving, etc.;
- remind you to pee every hour or so;
- be your advocate and speak up for you as needed.

Kieran's Birth Day

Christy and Angelo had planned to have lots of support for the birth of their first child, and appreciated all of it when labor turned out to be long and slow. Christy labored at home for 17 hours, encouraged by her aunt, her midwives, and Angelo. She spent some time walking in her yard, relaxing in the bathtub, and sitting upright while her support people rubbed her back and helped her relax. Eventually they went to the hospital where Christy had some medication for pain relief, and baby Kieran was born 7 hours later, weighing 9 lbs. ½ oz.

Do You Want a Doula?

As well as a person to provide medical care, you might consider arranging for a doula or another support person to help you through labor. A doula is not a doctor or midwife, but a trained labor support person who usually meets with the woman and her partner during pregnancy, then stays with her throughout labor and birth. The doula doesn't provide medical care, but simply supports the mother and her partner. She could be a childbirth educator or student midwife; other doulas may be members of DONA (Doulas of North America).

A doula isn't a good idea just for someone with no other support people. Alisa, for example, had her family doctor, her husband and her mother (also a doctor) with her when her baby was born, but she says, "I would testify to the *necessity* of professional labor support in addition to the presence of loved ones and family members." She labored at home with her two doulas until about two hours before her daughter was born. "This arrangement was perfect for me. With the indispensable help of our doulas, we had a peaceful, unmedicated (though very intense) birth."

If you are a single mother, or have a partner who is not planning to be part of labor and birth, a doula can be even more important. Lisa, a single mother, says that finding a doula "was the best decision I made." She met with this support person during her pregnancy and says that "by the time I was ready to give birth, I felt empowered. Even though my labor took 36 hours, I don't consider my birthing experience one of the hardest things I have done, but one of the best and certainly the most rewarding." She spent most of her labor at home, but went to the hospital seven hours before her son was born. Lisa delivered in a squatting position and had no medication. "The whole experience was so positive."

Isn't labor support the father's or partner's role? Will the doula come between the husband and wife? Susan Martensen, one of the founders of LSAR (Labour Support Association and Registry) says, "The doula doesn't replace the partner but helps him. He knows more about his wife, and can provide the love and closeness, but the doula knows more about labor and birth, and techniques that are helpful. Fathers often tell us how glad they were that the doula was there."

Research on doulas and having a support person during labor has been positive. Women who had doulas with them tended to have shorter labors, fewer forceps deliveries and fewer Caesarean sections. However, these studies were done in hospital settings where the stress and anxiety levels were quite high, and the results may not apply to all laboring women.

However, it's natural for people to want support and companionship during any stressful or challenging experience. The women quoted above were less concerned about whether having doulas shortened their labors, and more interested in the added confidence and comfort they felt because of the support they received.

birth, and many will allow other labor support people to be there as well. Some hospitals allow only one person, but women sometimes want to have more than one. As Nazreen says, "I had a long, tough labor, and I don't know if I could have gotten through it without my husband, my mother and my sister all with me. They took turns resting or napping and I always had someone to walk with me and rub my back."

A recent study looked at labor support given by people with specific training and experience. It found that mothers who had labor support from other women who had learned techniques for coping with the pain of labor used less medication and had fewer epidurals than mothers who had labor partners simply providing reassurance and emotional support.

Perhaps the best situation is when a woman has both the loving support of her partner as well as the expertise of a trained labor support woman, or doula. (See sidebar, "Do You Want a Doula?")

The Evidence About . . .
HOSPITAL ROUTINES AND LABOR SUPPORT

Research has found no benefits to giving enemas to women in labor or to shaving their pubic hair.

The benefits or hazards of using an electronic fetal monitor for 20 minutes on every woman when she arrives at the hospital have not yet been researched.

Not allowing women to eat or drink during labor does not guarantee protection against inhaling food or stomach acid in the event of surgery, and can have negative effects.

When women can choose to be upright and walking during labor, their labors are shorter and less painful.

Support from partners and others can lead to shorter labors requiring less pain-relieving medication.

19

How Is the Baby Doing? Assessing the Baby During Labor

Shirley was relaxing on the couch and watching TV with her husband when labor started. "I couldn't believe how close the contractions were right from the start," she said. "After about 10 contractions, my water broke—right there in the living room—and then things got even more painful."

The intensity of the contractions scared her, but she was also worried about her baby. Was this fast-moving labor as stressful for the baby as it was for her? Shirley was comforted when her midwife arrived and listened to the baby's heartbeat with a stethoscope. "Baby's doing fine," the midwife reassured her.

When you go into labor, either the midwife who attends you at home or the nurses in the hospital will frequently listen to the baby's heart. The baby's heart rate is the main indicator of its well-being during labor. The goal is to detect any problems—signaled by changes in the baby's heart rate patterns—that might indicate that the baby is not getting enough oxygen. The baby who has a problem is often described as being "in distress."

With everything that is going on in labor, keeping an eye on the baby's well-being is important. Ideally, this monitoring process will be selective enough that it won't produce many "false alarms" and subject a lot of babies to interventions they don't need, yet sensitive enough to identify all babies who are in distress. We also want to be sure that the interventions done to help those babies in distress are actually improving the outcome.

Heart Rate Monitoring

Intermittent Monitoring: Spot Checks throughout Labor

There are several different ways to keep an eye on the baby's heart rate for signs of stress during labor. The most common method is intermittently listening to the baby's heart, either with a special stethoscope or with a hand-held ultrasound monitor.

How often should the nurse or other caregiver check the baby? Every hospital will have its own policy, but a common routine is for the nurse to listen for one minute every 30 minutes in early labor, every 15 minutes in active labor and every five minutes when the mother begins to push the baby out. The nurse will count the number of beats per minute she hears and write that on the mother's chart.

In practice, there are wide variations in how long the nurse listens and how frequently she makes these checks. If the labor and delivery department is very busy, the nurse may need to spend more time with a mother who is having some difficulties, and another mother, where labor is going well, will be checked less frequently.

The baby is considered to be in fetal distress if the heart rate is faster than 160 to 180 beats per minute, or slower than 100 to 120 beats per minute, for any length of time. It is also a concern if the baby's heartbeat is very irregular.

Researchers have assumed that listening to the baby's heartbeat in labor is beneficial, but there have been no studies comparing listening to the baby with not listening. It's unlikely that this research will ever be done, since listening to the baby's heart is now such an accepted part of care during labor. There have also been no studies to see if there are better outcomes depending on how often these checks of the baby's heart rate are done. (This is why various hospitals have different routines—no particular schedule has been established as "the best.")

Continuous Monitoring: The High-Tech Approach

In the 1970s, a new machine was developed that could listen to and record the baby's heartbeat continuously throughout labor: the electronic fetal monitor (EFM).

There are two ways of doing continuous monitoring. With external monitoring, a belt is strapped around the mother's abdomen and holds an ultrasound paddle in place to record the baby's heartbeat. A second belt picks up the contractions. For internal monitoring, the membranes must be ruptured. If they have not ruptured before this point, the doctor will need to rupture them before putting on the internal monitor. A clip is inserted through the vagina and cervix and attached to the baby's scalp.

With either type, the heart rate is then recorded on a monitor positioned beside the mother's bed and attached by wires to the belt or clip. Usually, the machine beeps each time the baby's heart beats, and shows a constantly changing number giving the baby's heart rate (you might see 138, 140, 144, 145, 142 and so on). The other belt records the contractions. A continuous record of the baby's heartbeat and the contractions of the uterus is printed out on a long strip of graph paper.

Continuous monitoring is technically much more difficult than just having a nurse press a stethoscope against the mother's belly. With external monitoring, whenever the fetus or mother moves the signal may be lost and the paddle must be readjusted. Sometimes it is the mother's heart rate that is being recorded, rather than the baby's, and this can worry everyone because it's normally much slower than the baby's. Once the baby starts to move down into the birth canal, it becomes quite challenging to position the paddle over the baby's heart, especially if the mother is upright or moving around to find a comfortable position for birth.

Elisabeth recalls, "Every time I moved, the monitor's beep of the baby's heart would get really faint. I'd panic, my husband would panic, and I'd try not to move any more. Then the nurse would calmly readjust the belts and it would be fine—until I moved again. After a while, my husband asked them to turn off the sound, and that helped."

Noor found the monitor restrictive. "They wanted me in one position and I just wasn't comfortable. I wanted to be able to move around more. Then, at one point, the nurse came in and said, 'Have you stopped having contractions?' I'd somehow moved the belt again so it wasn't recording the contractions at all. She was quite annoyed with me about that."

When internal monitoring is used, there is a risk of the scalp clip coming off the baby's scalp. This can cause a momentary panic because it looks as though the baby's heartbeat has stopped. There is also a higher risk of infection when a scalp clip is used. This may be not just from the clip itself, but from the fact that the clip is often used in long or complicated labors where there have been lots of vaginal exams and other interventions.

Which Type of Monitoring Is Better?

Even when continuous monitoring is working well, there are concerns. Doctors interpret the patterns they see in different ways, and what one doctor thinks is a sign of a baby in distress, another doctor may think is perfectly fine. There are no hard and fast rules; the more years that continuous monitoring has been used, the more researchers have realized that what they thought was an abnormal pattern may be normal for many babies.

Many women find continuous monitoring uncomfortable. It makes it impossible for them to walk around and prevents them from moving into positions that might be more comfortable. But the most important issue is whether continuous monitoring can improve outcomes for the baby.

Large clinical trials (including 17,000 women) have compared the outcomes for mothers and babies of using a stethoscope to check on the baby intermittently or of continuous monitoring with an EFM during labor.

> The Society of Obstetricians and Gynaecologists of Canada currently recommends intermittent monitoring of the baby during labor rather than routine, continuous monitoring.

The results were disappointing for those who had high hopes for EFM: Caesarean section rates and rates of forceps and vacuum deliveries were all significantly higher in the continuously monitored group. Outcomes for the babies, however, were exactly the same in both groups. The number of fetal deaths, low Apgar scores and admissions to special care nurseries was the same in both the continuously and the intermittently monitored group. There was one small difference: when continuous monitoring with fetal scalp sampling (see the next page) was used, fewer newborns had seizures than in the intermittently monitored group. These seizures were not associated with any ongoing problems. Long-term follow-up showed no difference in the rates of cerebral palsy between the two groups. *The inescapable conclusion is that continuous monitoring increases interventions—Caesarean section, forceps and vacuum delivery—with no benefit to the baby.*

If continuous monitoring is used at your hospital, you can refuse it and ask that a nurse check your baby intermittently instead. This will also allow you to walk around and change position during labor more easily.

What about the 20-minute Initial "Strip"?

At many hospitals, women who arrive in labor are hooked up to the fetal monitor for a period of time, usually 15 to 20 minutes. After this, the mother may have the belts removed and be permitted to walk around or change position.

This brief use of continuous monitoring has not been studied enough to identify any risks or benefits. There is no reason to believe that it is any more helpful than longer periods of continuous monitoring, which have been shown not to improve outcomes for the baby.

Andrea says, "I was only supposed to be on the monitor for 20 minutes, but then things got busy and nobody came back to take it off. I was having back labor and the position I was in made it worse. I wish I'd had the confidence to just take the belts off myself and get up, but I kept waiting for someone to come and tell me it was okay."

You can decline to have the 20-minute strip done. Just tell the nurse you have decided against it.

Fetal Scalp Sampling

Another method used to "keep an eye on the baby" is fetal scalp sampling.

When the baby is not getting enough oxygen, the pH (a measure of the acidity of the baby's blood) decreases. By taking a sample of blood from the baby's scalp, your doctor can measure the pH level and determine if the baby is in distress.

This is a technically tricky procedure. It's most easily done with the mother lying on her back with her legs up in stirrups (a position that can actually *cause* fetal distress). A special speculum is put into the vagina so the doctor can see and feel the cervix and the baby's head. The membranes must be ruptured. The spot to be sampled must be wiped completely clean of all fluid and any of the mother's blood before the scalp is pricked to get the blood sample. Then pressure must be kept on the spot to make sure the baby doesn't keep bleeding. Since fetal scalp sampling is awkward and

time-consuming, it is usually done only if heart rate changes suggest the baby is in distress.

A fetal scalp pH of 7.2 or above suggests that the baby is fine, and that no intervention is necessary. A fetal scalp pH of below 7.2 suggests that the baby is in distress.

This gives three possible methods of assessing the baby in labor: intermittent monitoring, continuous monitoring and scalp sampling if the baby's heart rate suggests it might be in distress. When researchers compared these procedures, the results were:

- Caesarean sections, forceps and vacuum extractors were used most often with continuous monitoring, less often when fetal scalp sampling was added and least often when the baby was intermittently monitored.
- Babies did equally well in all three groups, with one small exception. When fetal scalp sampling was used, fewer babies had seizures during the newborn period. These seizures were not associated with any long-term problems.

Stimulation of the Fetus to Assess Fetal Heart Rate

If the baby's heart rate speeds up in response to contractions or movement, this is considered to be a positive indicator that baby is doing well.

Some researchers have noted that sound and touch can also cause the baby's heart rate to speed up. Studies have been done comparing the baby's reaction to sound (using a noise-making device placed on the mother's abdomen) and touch (using pressure or gentle pinching of the baby's scalp). The researchers also did fetal scalp sampling on these babies. They found that if the baby responded to sound or touch with a faster heartbeat, the fetal scalp sampling result would be good as well.

More research is needed, but this looks like a promising—and much simpler—way to monitor babies in labor. Only those who do not respond to the sound or touch would need scalp sampling to further assess the possibility of distress.

If the Baby Is in Distress, What Then?

When the baby's heart rate drops and stays low, the doctor or midwife will usually do a vaginal examination to see if the umbilical cord has slipped into the vagina and is being compressed by the baby's head. This vaginal exam will also indicate how close the woman is to giving birth.

The simplest step to take when the baby appears to be in distress is to change position. If you are lying on your back, even when the head of the bed is elevated, you are compressing the aorta and vena cava (the major artery and vein of the body) and reducing blood flow to the fetus. You can try lying on your side, which can dramatically increase the circulation to the baby. Changing position may also improve heart rate problems caused by pressure on the umbilical cord.

If the mother is given extra oxygen (in a mask she can hold over her nose and mouth) the baby will get more oxygen as well.

If the mother is receiving oxytocin by IV to stimulate the labor and the baby shows signs of distress, the oxytocin should be discontinued immediately.

If the mother's blood pressure drops, the baby may show signs of distress. This frequently happens when an epidural or spinal anesthetic is given. The drop in blood pressure can be prevented by giving the mother intravenous fluids to increase her blood volume before administering the epidural or spinal.

The mother's blood pressure can also drop if she changes position suddenly (sitting up or standing up quickly, for example). She is more likely to experience this if she has been given narcotic painkillers such as Demerol. Try not to get up quickly when you are in labor; if you find yourself feeling faint, lie down on your side. Drinking frequently during labor also helps to reduce this problem. If you are throwing up repeatedly and not able to keep liquids down, you might consider having an IV put in to give you more fluids.

If these steps haven't improved the baby's heart rate, the next step is to just get the baby born. If labor has progressed far enough, that can mean use of a vacuum extractor or forceps to deliver the baby quickly. If the cervix is not fully dilated, or if the baby is not low enough in the birth canal to make vacuum or forceps possible, a Caesarean section will be recommended.

This can be a frightening time for parents. Hannah remembers her labor as "overwhelming. I was going too slowly at first, so they gave me oxytocin in an IV to get things moving. But before long, the contractions got really strong, and then the baby went into distress. We could all see it on the monitor, his heart rate just dropped, and it was just beep...beep...beep. My husband started yelling at the nurse to 'do something.'

"They stopped the oxytocin and had me roll onto my side. But it didn't help. There was still that ominous, slow beeping. The doctor shook his head and told me we had to do a C-section. They gave me a general anesthetic because it was faster, and when I came around again I didn't even know if the baby was okay. I was afraid to ask. I think it was even worse for Chad, waiting outside the room to hear the news. But the news was good. Mark's first Apgar score was low, but then he was fine, and he's doing great now."

Other Approaches for Fetal Distress

Clinical trials to assess other methods of managing fetal distress have been too small to allow any conclusions other than that they look promising and need larger trials.

When there is only a small amount of amniotic fluid (called oligohydramnios), there is more opportunity for the umbilical cord to be compressed and the oxygen supply to the baby to be decreased. The volume of fluid can be increased by putting a little tubing through the vagina into the uterus and infusing solution through it into the uterus. Small studies have shown improved fetal heart rates and healthier babies, without increasing the rate of Caesarean section. (See also Chapter 27, Problems with the Amniotic Fluid.)

Terbutaline is a drug that relaxes smooth muscles and is used to stop premature labor. Intravenous terbutaline has also been used to reduce signs of fetal distress when there is a delay before the baby can be delivered. Studies have shown better outcomes for babies, but these trials have been very small.

Piracetam and pyridoxine are drugs used to "treat" the fetus to prevent damage from fetal distress. Small studies appear promising.

The Evidence About...
ASSESSING THE BABY DURING LABOR

When continuous monitoring is used during labor, more babies will be delivered by Caesarean section, forceps or vacuum extractors, with no improvement in outcome.

When fetal scalp sampling is added to this monitoring, the intervention rate is lower.

When babies are monitored intermittently, the intervention rate is lowest of all, and the babies do just as well as with the other methods.

Intermittent monitoring is recommended by both the Society of Obstetricians and Gynaecologists of Canada and the authors of *Effective Care in Pregnancy and Childbirth*.

While prompt delivery is the usual method for dealing with fetal distress, changing the mother's position or giving her oxygen also may be helpful.

The story of continuous electronic fetal monitoring should serve as a cautionary tale: monitors were readily accepted and quickly pressed into routine use at many hospitals before their value had been tested by research. As a result, many women experienced unnecessary Caesarean sections and other interventions. Any new procedures should be thoroughly researched before being introduced into routine practice.

20

Coping with Pain in Labor

How Much Does Labor Hurt?

As soon as you knew you were pregnant, you probably started to wonder what labor would be like and how you would cope with the pain. Reading books and seeing videos doesn't really tell you what it will feel like, and as you talk to other women you will discover that everyone's experience is unique.

Sylvia's labor, which took about eight hours, she remembers as being "easy." "Except for the last 20 minutes or so, I would describe the contractions as being like strong menstrual cramps. It wasn't as bad as I had expected, and it really fooled the nurse because she thought I was a long way from delivering."

Pam remembers being absolutely terrified of the pain of labor all through her pregnancy. "When labor started, I kept telling myself not to get too upset, because I knew it was going to get worse. I paced around the house saying, 'Keep calm, it's going to get worse.' Finally I went to the hospital. The nurse told me I was 8 cm dilated. I asked her when it was going to

get really bad. She laughed and said it was just about as bad as it was going to get right now, and just to keep doing what I was doing. I walked and muttered 'Keep calm, keep calm'...right up until I pushed the baby out."

Angela had a three-hour labor and says that almost from the first contraction "the pain was unbearable. The first pains were so awful that I woke my husband and we went to the hospital right away. The contractions became even more intense in the car. I was crying uncontrollably by the time we got to the hospital.

"We had to wait in the admitting department for the clerk to find my form, before we went to the birthing suite. In the birthing suite, as soon as the nurse heard that my contractions had started not even an hour ago, she obviously just thought I was hysterical—which I was! The department was really busy—people kept popping in to do things and then leaving again. The nurse went through this whole questionnaire. After a while, an intern came and saw me and of course asked most of the same questions. The lab came and took my blood. During it all, I was crying in between the contractions and just about screaming during them. My back never stopped aching, and during the contractions I felt like I was being ripped apart.

"Then I started to feel like I had to go to the bathroom. I knew women got diarrhea in labor, and I thought that was coming. I went into the bathroom and I could hear this grunting noise. It was me. Then the nurse rushed in—I guess she heard me—and before I knew what was happening I was on the bed and my doctor was there and the baby was born."

Even though people were with Angela to do particular procedures, she felt alone most of the time. She thinks now her panic was not just from the pain itself. "All the stories I had heard said a first labor takes about 12 hours. I was only two hours into labor and I couldn't stand it. It never occurred to me I was going to be quicker than average. I just kept thinking, 'I can't bear this pain for 10 more hours.' My husband didn't have a clue what to do—he was as frantic as I was."

Were Angela and Sylvia and Pam all feeling the same thing? Why is one labor more painful than another? Why is one labor longer than another? And why does one treatment to relieve pain work well for one woman and do nothing for the next? There are more questions about pain in labor than there are answers.

The pain of labor is different from most pain, in that it does not result from an injury or disease, or signal that something is wrong. It's a "working" pain, pain that occurs normally as the uterus does its job of opening the cervix and getting the baby out. But how *much* pain is "normal" or tolerable is not something that can be measured.

Individual women have different experiences of labor, and they also have different expectations and attitudes. Some women take

for granted that labor will be painful. Alice said, "All those muscles that had to hold the baby in for nine months had to open up completely in a few hours. It hurt about as much as I figured it should." Other women are equally clear that they are not willing to go through a painful labor. Lisa told her doctor at her first prenatal appointment, "I want an epidural as early as I can have it. I have no intention of suffering."

Do women who believe that pain in labor is normal find it easier to put up with? Do women who believe that pain in labor is something that needs to be controlled or relieved actually find the pain worse? These are questions that don't have any answers, and it is hard to imagine designing research that would answer them.

Research on Pain Relief

The perfect pain reliever in labor would need to have many qualities:

- It should relieve the pain.
- It shouldn't have any negative effects on the mother such as vomiting, dizziness, being unable to empty her bladder or feeling as though she is "watching" her labor but not participating in it.
- It shouldn't have any negative effects on the labor, such as making it take longer, taking away the urge to push or making it more likely that the woman will bleed too much. It shouldn't make it more likely that the woman will need a forceps delivery or a Caesarean section.
- It shouldn't have any negative effects on the baby, such as making its heartbeat slow or causing breathing problems after the birth.

Unfortunately, most of the pain-relieving

Tips for Labor Pain Relief

- Preparation is important, since most people fear the unknown. Knowing what happens in labor and why will help you to feel confident.
- Slow, relaxed breathing is helpful.
- Listen to music; if you give birth in a hospital, bring your own tape or CD and player.
- Try water therapy—take a shower, sit in a tub, try a whirlpool.
- Gentle massage can be relaxing, although some laboring women don't like to be touched.
- Walking around not only shortens labor but makes it more comfortable.
- If you decide to sit up in bed, change positions frequently.
- For back labor, try kneeling on all fours, leaning against a table, lying on one side or straddling a chair or toilet seat backwards. Also try strong counterpressure against your back, or applying ice or a heating pad.
- Eat if you're hungry and take sips of juice or ginger ale.
- Empty your bladder frequently, even if you don't feel like you need to go.
- Try imagining a peaceful setting or focusing on images of "opening up."
- Low moaning noises are a good way to release tension.
- Having a constant companion is extremely valuable. In case labor is long, it helps to have more than one support person.

divided into two big groups—those that involve the use of drugs and those that don't.

Drug-Free Approaches to Easing Labor Pain

Breathing Techniques

Using specific patterns of breathing in and out is probably the first technique that comes to mind when we talk about pain relief in labor. It was the central focus of most of the earlier prenatal classes, and some childbirth educators have written entire books about different types of breathing for different stages of labor.

Using breathing patterns is intended to help you focus your concentration on something other than the pain of the contractions. This distraction, it is hoped, will help you relax and be less aware of painful sensations. Does it work? Some women find the breathing techniques extremely helpful, while others find they don't help at all.

While breathing patterns themselves have not been researched, studies have been done to see if prenatal classes reduce the need for pain-relieving drugs during labor. When these studies were done, prenatal classes spent a great deal of time teaching breathing techniques, and the studies did find that the classes reduced the need for medications to relieve pain in labor.

Melanie felt that the breathing techniques she learned helped her: "I just used the basic, slow breathing almost all the way through. It helped me to relax and gave me something to concentrate on during contractions, and I know it made the contractions more bearable."

Suzanne, on the other hand, didn't find the techniques helpful at all. "I did the breathing in the beginning, but after a while it all fell apart. I was moaning more than anything else,

treatments that really take pain away can affect the labor, the mother and the baby.

Pain-relieving techniques are generally

Adrienne Leong

and I couldn't remember what I was supposed to be doing. It just didn't work for me."

Visualization

Women who use visualization during labor might create mental images of a relaxing setting or a peaceful memory, and usually practice this in advance with their partners. Other images used during visualization are those that remind the mother of the cervix dilating and the baby coming out, such as a flower opening.

Visualization has not been researched in the context of labor, but has proven useful in some other areas, such as sports.

Prenatal Classes

Attendance at any prenatal classes (no matter what the content) has been consistently shown to reduce the amount of painkillers used during labor.

Does this mean that the pain was less, 161 or does it mean that education about labor helped women to accept pain as normal? Does it mean that learning about the complications of drugs made women more ready to tolerate pain rather than to use drugs or does it mean that women who decide to take prenatal classes are less likely to use drugs anyway? We don't know.

Freedom of Movement in Labor

When women are given the freedom to move and choose any positions they want for labor, most prefer to be sitting, standing or walking most of the time. When women choose to lie down, it's usually during very early labor (when "resting up" is a good idea) or at the very end of labor. Women who are experiencing "back labor" (feeling most of the pain and pressure in their lower backs) will often get down on their hands and knees, lean against a chair or the bed or sit on the toilet.

Deanna danced through much of her labor.

What Women Say about Their Partners and Labor Support

As her partner, you can't control the course of her labor or take away the pain. You might even feel that you really aren't much use. But chances are, you will help her more than you know. Here's what some women remember about their partners' support:

- "He timed the contractions so he could warn me when another one was about to start and I'd get into a comfortable position before it hit."
- "He really supported me physically. I walked around through most of my labor and every time a contraction hit I'd lean on him. And when the baby was born, I was squatting and he held me up under my arms."
- "He held the basin for me to throw up in and never said a word."
- "When I felt like I couldn't go on, he held my face in his hands and made me look at him and said, 'Breathe now, breathe, breathe,' and just kept me going through those really hard contractions."
- "He was just there for me. He held my hand and whenever I looked at him, he'd smile and nod. That was so important to me."
- "I had a Caesarean and a general anesthetic, but when I opened my eyes again he was standing there holding the baby and tears were running down his face. He said, 'You did it, you did it,' and I felt wonderful despite the surgery."
- "I couldn't have done it without him."

"I felt it really helped me to keep moving. I played the tape I had prepared when I was pregnant, and walked around the room, swaying to the music. I'd hum loudly—okay, sometimes it was moaning—during the contractions. It all helped."

Ann gave birth to her son on a beautiful spring day in May. "We dropped the older two children off at my sister's and then went to walk in the park. I spent about four hours there, walking along the pathways and enjoying the sunshine. I was surprised at how relaxed I felt. Eventually the contractions got strong enough that we decided to go to the hospital. Even now, every time I drive past that park, I remember walking there on that gorgeous day and waiting for my son to be born."

Norah spent a lot of her labor on the toilet. "It worked best if I sat backwards so I could rest my arms and head on the tank. Plus, I liked that it was cool, because I was really sweating at that point. Afterwards, my midwife said she was a bit worried that I was going to give birth right on the toilet, but I did move onto the bed when I felt like pushing."

Walking during labor is linked to shorter labor, less medication for pain and less fetal distress. Yet, women in labor in hospital have often been kept in bed for no particular reason. The introduction of continuous fetal monitoring and IVs made it more difficult for the mother to move around or get out of bed. Skimpy hospital gowns embarrass some women and discourage them from walking around—so bring a generous bathrobe, your own nightgown or an oversized T-shirt from home to wear.

Sometimes women have been so conditioned by years of movies and TV shows that show women lying in bed as they labored, or are so intimidated by the hospital environment, that they find it difficult to know what positions or ways of moving would be most comfortable for them. Caregivers and support people can help with suggestions ("Let's go for a walk down the hall" or "Why don't you sit up for a while?").

As labor progresses and the baby moves down into the pelvis, a position that was helpful and comfortable may quickly become painful, and the mother will need to move again. The mother is the best judge of what feels most comfortable to her at any particular point in her labor.

Touch

Touch reminds the laboring woman that she is not alone, that there are people there who care for her and that she has support and help close by. No wonder a gentle touch can be so relaxing! A hot water bottle on the back or a cold cloth pressed to a sweaty forehead give not just physical relief, but a sense of being cared for.

The variations of touch are infinite. It can be as simple as holding hands or letting her lean against you during a contraction. Suzanne describes walking around her apartment with her husband David in early labor: "We were just strolling around, and then when the contraction would hit, I stopped walking. I didn't even have to say anything. David would put his arms around me and I'd rest my head on his shoulder and stay in that position until the contraction went away."

Massage is another form of touch that can be helpful in labor. It can be used to relax tense shoulders, arms or legs. Some women like to have their abdomens massaged lightly during contractions. If the mother is experiencing a lot of back pain, she may like very firm massaging of her lower back and buttocks, or counterpressure (firm, direct pressure) against her lower back. Since a long labor can mean many hours of massaging, it's a good idea to bring powder or lotion to use on the mother's skin to prevent irritation.

Mariana had both her husband and a doula walking with her in labor. When a contraction arrived, she'd lean against her husband and he would massage her shoulders. The doula would rub her lower back, where she was feeling increasing pressure. "The massaging helped so much," Mariana says.

Rita says, "I think the most important thing is for your husband to pay attention to you. I could hardly talk once the contractions got strong, and I remember one time saying 'Back!' to John so he would rub my back, but he wasn't paying attention, so he didn't do anything. When the contraction finally went away I yelled at him."

Partners and support people also need to be aware that massaging or other touch that has been helpful at one point in labor may suddenly become annoying and uncomfortable. The mother may only be able to say "Stop" or "No" at that point, so the partner needs to be alert.

Massage and other forms of touch have not been systematically researched, but it is difficult to see how they could have any risks. Since women almost universally speak positively about it, touch will continue to be an important part of pain relief in labor.

Immersion in Water

During the "walking-around" process, many laboring women find themselves—like divining rods—heading for water. Baths, whirlpools and showers are often comforting and relaxing during labor, and increasing numbers of hospitals are adding these facilities to their labor and delivery units. Women with back labor sometimes like to stand with the shower aimed at their lower backs. Other women find that sitting or lying in warm water—in either an ordinary bath or pool or a whirlpool—is very relaxing and reduces their awareness of pain.

"One reason I chose this hospital," says Inez, "was the Jacuzzi. I loved feeling the water swirling over me. It was like being massaged by several people at once, and it got me through the worst part of labor."

Some mothers end up giving birth in the bath or pool (either intentionally or because they find it too difficult to get out of the water when the moment of birth arrives). While this has not been extensively researched, no higher complication rates have been noted so far. A few individual case reports suggest that it is safest to keep the water at around body temperature, so the woman does not get overheated, and that the baby should be lifted from the water as soon as it is born.

Acupuncture

Acupuncture consists of the placement of needles in specific points, and then stimulation through those needles either by twirling them or sometimes through an electric current. No controlled trials of acupuncture for pain relief during labor have been published, although it is used effectively for more chronic pain.

Acupressure is "acupuncture without needles." It consists of deep pressure on specific acupuncture points. No trials of its effectiveness in labor have been published.

Injection of Sterile Water

Controlled trials have shown dramatic relief from back pain in labor by injecting 0.1 ml (0.003 fl oz) of sterile water just under the skin of the lower back at four specific spots around the sacrum (the very bottom bone in the spine). This simple measure has no known complications. The reason it relieves the pain is not known, but it might be the same mechanism that makes acupuncture work for pain relief.

Since sterile water is normally available in hospitals, you could ask your doctor about this if you are interested in trying it.

Hypnosis

When people have been hypnotized, they are temporarily more relaxed, more open to suggestion and more able to change the perception of pain. Theoretically, it would be an ideal painkiller during labor.

Hypnosis can be used in either of two ways: the woman can be hypnotized during her pregnancy, and left with the post-hypnotic suggestion that the sensations of labor will be powerful and intense, but not painful; or the woman can be taught to hypnotize herself and enter a trance during labor to reduce awareness of pain.

However, one clinical trial of hypnosis during labor found no difference in drug use between the hypnotized and the non-hypnotized groups. The length of labor in the hypnosis group was much longer. Another study found shorter labors in the hypnosis group.

Music

Music during labor can be a pleasant distraction that can help the mother to picture relaxing surroundings and images. Music can also create a cheerful atmosphere for the partner, the support people and the staff caring for her. As well, music can block out unpleasant "hospital" sounds (such as the woman screaming in the next room).

The specific use of soothing music between contractions and "white sound" during contractions, at a volume controlled by the mother, has been researched in small clinical trials. The mothers listening to music reported less pain and also used fewer drugs during labor.

Stephanie brought a tape she and her husband had put together to the hospital. "I think it made us all feel calmer. I will always remember my doctor and my husband singing along to the tape while we waited for me to have another pushing contraction. I don't know if it really relieved pain, but I definitely felt more relaxed."

Transcutaneous Electrical Nerve Stimulation (TENS)

TENS uses a portable box containing a battery-powered generator of electrical impulses. Electrodes are taped to the back and the electrical impulses are transmitted to the skin of the back via wires attached to the box, resulting in a buzzing or tingling sensation. The woman can adjust the intensity of these impulses during contractions. The electrical impulses are intended to "block" the pain sensations.

More clinical trials have been done on TENS than on any other non-drug method of pain relief. Their results are almost contradictory—results show that women like TENS and report favorably on it, yet report a higher incidence of intense pain. The use of TENS does not reduce the use of drugs during labor.

If a woman plans to use TENS, she must rent the equipment and learn to use it before labor begins. Women who select this method may be those who anticipate both that the pain of labor will be severe and that it will need treatment.

How We Think about Pain in Labor

Do non-drug therapies for pain relief "work"? There isn't any objective way of assessing their effectiveness.

If "working" means do women use them and like them, the answer is an emphatic "yes."

If "working" means do women who use them use fewer drugs during labor, the answer is "we don't know for sure, but probably not."

The 1997 edition of *Williams Obstetrics*, a standard textbook, devotes 20 pages to pain relief in labor. Of those 20 pages, only three paragraphs discuss non-drug methods. One of these paragraphs is interesting: "When motivated women have been prepared for childbirth, pain during labor has been found to be diminished by one third. The presence of a supportive spouse or other family member, of conscientious labor attendants, and of a considerate obstetrician who instills confidence, contribute greatly to accomplishing this goal of pain relief."

The small space allotted to non-drug techniques in this textbook sends a clear message—that doctors don't really think these methods are important. The textbook gives lip service to the idea that these methods are useful and have been shown to reduce pain, but then doesn't bother to describe the methods or how they might become part of standard care.

This message is often reinforced in hospital. The doctor's last words as he leaves the laboring woman's room are often, "I'll leave an order for a shot of Demerol when you want it." The nurse making her regular blood pressure check often bustles in on the couple who are managing each contraction with back massage and some groaning and says, "Just ring when you want your epidural."

Is this just making sure that choices are available, which is a stated goal of family-centered maternity care? Or does this undermine the normalcy of labor? Every time a mother is reminded about the availability of medication during labor, it reinforces the idea that "something should be done" about the pain.

How important is suggestion in pain relief? Even using the phrase pain relief suggests that labor pain—which is, after all, a universal and normal experience—*needs* to be relieved. Perhaps the methods described as non-drug pain relievers don't actually diminish the pain but help the mother to cope with it. That's equally valuable.

Clarifying Your Feelings about Pain and Medications in Labor

Penny Simkin, who is a doula and childbirth educator, has developed a table that you can use to clarify your feelings about the use of pain medication in labor. The chart also provides a "reality check" on your expectations, and will help you discuss and plan for the kind of labor support you may need.

Look down the middle column to see the description that most closely fits your feelings, then tell your partner, "I think I'm a +3" (or whatever number you have chosen). Your partner can then look across to the right-hand column for tips about helping you during labor.

The Number	What It Means	Your Partner, Doula or Caregiver Can Help You By
+10	I do not want to feel anything in labor. I want anesthesia before labor begins.	Explaining to you why this is not possible or safe.
+9	I have great fear of labor pain. I believe I cannot cope. I have to depend on the staff to take away my pain.	Doing the same as for +10 above. Teaching you some simple comfort techniques for early labor. Reassuring you that someone will always be there to help you
+7	I want anesthesia as soon in labor as the doctor will allow or before labor becomes painful.	Doing the same as +9 above. Making sure the staff knows you want early anesthesia. Making sure you know the procedures and the potential risks.
+5	I want epidural anesthesia in active labor (4–5 cm [1.6–2 in]). I am willing to try to cope until then, perhaps with narcotic medications.	Encouraging you in your breathing and relaxation. Knowing and using other comfort measures. Suggesting medications when you are in active labor.

The Number	What It Means	Your Partner, Doula or Caregiver Can Help You By
+3	I want to use some medication but as little as possible. I plan to use self-help comfort measures for part of labor.	Doing the same as +5 above. Committing themselves to helping you reduce medication use. Helping you get medications when you decide you want them. Suggesting half doses of narcotics or a "light and late" epidural.
0	I have no opinion or preference. I will wait and see. (A rare attitude among pregnant women.)	Helping you become informed about labor pain, comfort measures and medications. Following your wishes during labor.
-3	I would like to avoid pain medication if I can, but if coping becomes difficult I'd feel like a "martyr" if I didn't get them.	Emphasizing coping techniques. Not suggesting that you take pain medications. Not trying to talk you out of them if you request them.
-5	I have a strong desire to avoid pain medications, mainly to avoid the side effects on me, my labor or my baby. I will accept medication for difficult or long labor.	Preparing for a very active support role. Practising comfort measures with you in class and at home. Not suggesting medications; if you ask, suggesting different comfort measures and more intense emotional support first. Helping you accept pain medications if you become exhausted or cannot benefit from support techniques and comfort measures.

Clarifying Your Feelings about Pain and Medications in Labor (continued)

The Number	What It Means	Your Partner, Doula or Caregiver Can Help You By
-7	I have a very strong desire for a natural birth, for personal gratification along with the benefits to my baby and my labor. I will be disappointed if I use medication.	Doing the same as -5 above. Encouraging you to enlist the support of your caregiver. Requesting a supportive nurse who can help with natural birth. Planning and rehearsing ways to get through painful or discouraging periods in labor. Prearranging a plan (e.g., a "last resort" code word) for letting them know if you have had enough and truly want medication.
-9	I want medication to be denied by my support team and the staff even if I beg for it.	Exploring with you the reasons for your feelings. Helping you see that they cannot deny you medication. Promising to help all they can but leaving the final decision to you.
-10	I do not want any medication no matter what happens, even a Cesarean.	Helping you to learn about complications that require medication and intervention.

Reprinted with the permission of Penny Simkin PT and Childbirth Graphics.

Medications for Labor Pain

There has been more research about drugs for pain relief in labor than any other pregnancy treatment. However, most of this research has been aimed at discovering which drug works best (with the research being financially supported by the drug company) and comparing one drug to another. Painkillers are rarely compared to non-drug methods, and little attention is paid to possible effects on mothers and babies.

The important question to ask is: What method will give good relief without harm to mother or baby?

Tranquilizers

Sedatives, tranquilizers and sleeping pills have been used either by mouth or by injection in early labor to help women relax, to lessen their anxious feelings and to help them sleep. They have no pain-killing effect at all. They can cross the placenta and cause the baby to be depressed at birth, meaning it will not breathe well or suck well, and may be limp until the drug has worn off.

Narcotics

Narcotics (Demerol is the most common) can provide very good pain relief, but only at doses that can cause side-effects in both mother and baby. Lower, safer doses will not relieve pain noticeably. Different narcotics last for different lengths of time—varying from two to four hours. Narcotics are given either by intramuscular injection or intravenously.

Side-effects in the mother may include nausea and vomiting, dizziness and a drop in blood pressure. Narcotics usually prevent food that is eaten from being digested; instead, the food just sits in the stomach, and may be vomited up even hours after it has been eaten. There is no convincing evidence that Demerol given in active labor makes labor longer.

Narcotics cross the placenta and can cause the baby to not breathe well at birth. If this happens, the baby may need to be given oxygen through a mask, or spend some time on a respirator. The baby can be given an injection of a narcotic antagonist, which will counteract the effect of the narcotic and improve the baby's breathing. The possibility of depressed breathing in the baby is unpredictable—many mothers have had full doses of Demerol close to delivery and their babies have not had any breathing problems at all.

In one study, babies of mothers who received narcotics in labor tended to have lower Apgar scores and to be less responsive to their parents immediately after birth than those who received a placebo.

Another study compared shots of Demerol given by the nurse with an arrangement in which the laboring woman could give herself a dose of Demerol through an intravenous. The results showed that the pain relief was better, and a lower dose of narcotic was used, when the woman gave the drug to herself as she needed it. The usefulness of this method is limited by the need for an intravenous with a special pump.

Amy was given Demerol in labor and remembers it with mixed emotions. "It did help the pain, but I felt like I was going to throw up the whole rest of the labor. The worst part was after the baby was born, because I felt sleepy and completely out of it. The nurse was trying to give me Andrew to hold, but I kept drifting off."

Nancy, on the other hand, felt that the short-acting narcotic she was given really helped. "I was 7 cm (2.8 in), but the labor was so painful, much more than I was expecting. My doctor suggested a shot and I said yes. In about 10 minutes the pain of the contractions was much less and I was napping in between them. I thought the labor had really slowed down, but my husband said the contractions were still coming about every three minutes. I totally lost track of time. Then I had a really painful contraction and I said 'this is wearing off' and the very next contraction I had to push. The pushing didn't hurt at all like the labor pains—that one shot was all I had for the whole labor. It was great."

Antinausea Drugs

Labor itself often causes women to feel nauseated and to vomit, and narcotics given for pain in labor cause nausea and vomiting as well. Drugs like Gravol can be given during labor to try to control nausea, and are often given at the same time as the injection of a narcotic. Antinausea drugs can, like narcotics, cause dizziness and sleepiness in the mother.

Inhaled Painkillers ("Gas")

Anesthetic gas (usually nitrous oxide) can be inhaled by the mother at a dose that does not put her to sleep but helps to relieve the pain of labor. This can be used during the first stage of labor, or during the bearing-down stage. It is usually administered by a mask that the woman holds on her face herself. The woman is awake and in control of the painkiller, which doesn't last long and is easily stopped by taking the mask away.

Its disadvantage is that the mask must be tightly on the face while the mother is breathing in for it to reach a level that will relieve pain, and this is often a claustrophobic sensation for the laboring woman. It does not give complete pain relief, and its effectiveness varies a lot from one woman to another, at least in part because many women find it difficult to use. It can cause nausea and vomiting.

No obvious side-effects on the baby have been noticed.

Donna tried this method and didn't like it: "It was hard for me to focus on getting the mask in the right position and breathing in deeply when I was also trying to relax and get through the contraction. I took about four breaths and then I just barely got the mask out of the way in time to throw up. Since I was feeling pretty queasy anyway, I really didn't need that."

Epidural Anesthesia

The epidural is probably the first thing that most women think of when they are asked about pain relief during labor. Since its introduction in the early 1970s, it has become very widely used, because it can provide complete relief from pain, yet the mother is still conscious and able to see her baby being born.

The drug used is a local anesthetic, the same anesthetic that is injected by the dentist to freeze your mouth for dental work or is injected by the doctor to freeze you before you have stitches. In an epidural, the local anesthetic is injected into the epidural space, which is in your back, just outside the spinal canal.

The epidural is put in by an anesthetist, a doctor who specializes in administering this kind of medication. First, an intravenous will be started, because having extra fluid in the mother's circulation helps to prevent a drop in blood pressure from the epidural. The mother will either lie on her side curled up or sit up with her chin on her chest so the anesthetist can get the needle into the epidural space and inject the drug. Usually a tiny tubing is left in place for more drug to be injected as needed—this is called a continuous epidural. The drug can be injected periodically, either as the freezing wears off and the mother needs it or on a regular schedule. Studies have shown that regularly scheduled doses of freezing (called top-ups) give better pain relief than waiting for the freezing to wear off and then topping up.

Epidural or spinal injection: The woman is asked to lie with her back rounded to increase the space between the bones of the spine.

Another arrangement is a pump that is attached to the catheter and pumps the anesthetic continuously into the epidural space.

The epidural gives extremely effective pain relief—in fact, most women feel nothing at all in the area that is "frozen." Eighty-five percent of women have complete relief of pain, and 12 percent have partial relief. For the 3 percent who do not get relief, sometimes taking the catheter out and doing the epidural all over again will work.

The epidural can be put in at any stage of labor. It can be given in very early labor without using any other form of pain relief, or it can be used just for the delivery. It can be used as the next step if narcotics do not provide enough pain relief.

Women in labor are occasionally told that it is "too late" to have an epidural. This is not really true, as an epidural can be put in at any time. In practical terms, though, starting the intravenous, getting the anesthetist to the labor and delivery department and putting in the epidural all take time. If, in the estimation of the nurse or the doctor, the woman is going to give birth within the next hour or so, she may be told that "it's too late."

There have been very few studies with only small numbers of women on the effects of epidural on the baby. In these studies, there was no difference in the fetal heart rate, or in passing meconium during labor, with epidural anesthetic. Epidural is less likely than narcotic painkillers to cause low five-minute Apgar scores or low umbilical artery pH. (Low Apgar and low pH indicate a depressed baby who needs to be resuscitated.) A single report on 18-month-old babies found no difference between epidural and non-epidural babies.

Unfortunately, the epidural does have side-effects on the mother, and on the labor. The first stage of labor tends to be longer with an epidural, and oxytocin tends to be used more frequently to speed up labors when an epidural has been given. Researchers have also found a tendency for the second stage of labor to be longer, and a substantial increase in forceps or vacuum delivery. There is also a slight increase in the incidence of Caesarean section with epidural anesthetic.

Epidural anesthetic almost always means that the mother will be in bed for the rest of the labor, because it temporarily weakens the muscles in her legs. Some anesthetists specialize in "walking epidurals," which provide pain relief with less effect on the muscles. However, this is not widely available, and in most hospitals the policy is that women who have an epidural are in bed for the rest of the labor.

Epidural anesthetic can cause a temporary drop in the mother's blood pressure, which can cause dizziness, nausea and vomiting. As well, the epidural frequently makes women shiver, occasionally violently, and even though this is not harmful, it is extremely unpleasant.

The combination of being in bed and the anesthetic itself often makes women unable to empty their bladders, so a urinary catheter is frequently used for the rest of the labor. This increases the risk of a bladder infection after delivery.

When the epidural is being put in, it is possible for the anesthetist to accidentally puncture the dura, the lining of the spinal cord. This means that the epidural anesthetic cannot be given, and can also lead to severe headache for several days.

Life-threatening complications of epidural are rare, probably from 1 in 5000 to 1 in 10,000.

Women's feelings about epidurals range from great enthusiasm to disappointment. Ruth Anne says, "In the small town where I had Cody, epidurals were rare. They had to call in an anesthetist specially, so they hardly ever did them unless you needed a Caesarean or something. My labor wasn't long, but it really hurt, and the shot the nurse gave me didn't help a bit. Then we moved to Toronto, and I had Jamie. I couldn't believe the difference. As soon as I got to the hospital, they offered me the epidural and I took it. It was like I wasn't even in labor—there was no pain at all, just the excitement of waiting for the baby. A few hours later, Jamie was delivered with forceps, and even when the doctor stitched me up I didn't feel a thing. If I have another baby, I'll definitely get the epidural again."

Daria was also glad she had the epidural, but was unhappy about some parts of it: "Frankly, once I had the epidural, it was boring. I was glad not to feel the pain any more, but it was like I wasn't there. The nurse came in, looked at the monitor, checked my blood pressure and went out again. My husband was put off by all the tubes—I had the epidural catheter in my back, an intravenous, a catheter in my bladder and the fetal monitor on my belly—and he spent most of the time in the waiting room watching TV."

For Danielle, the experience of having an epidural was less positive. "I really wanted to have a natural birth. My labor turned out to be very long, and towards the end I was really tired. The nurse kept asking me if I wanted the epidural now. I told her a couple of times that I didn't want it, I would try to keep going a little longer, and finally she said, 'You know, it's going to get worse.' That did it. I said I'd take the epidural.

"But as soon as it was in, I started to cry. It stopped the pain, but I felt so detached from the whole thing, it was more like watching a movie than really having a baby. The next day, I felt really angry at that nurse for pushing the epidural when she knew I didn't want it. I'm sure she was just trying to help, but that was how I felt."

The frequency with which epidurals are used has a lot more to do with how available they are than with variations in the amount of pain women are experiencing. Some hospitals have anesthetists on hand to provide epidurals for any woman who requests one; in other hospitals, an anesthetist must be called in and epidurals are reserved for Caesarean sections or forceps deliveries.

One community hospital experienced this when the anesthesiology staff changed their policy and became much less available. In one year, the rate of epidural use went from 75 percent to 30 percent. The women didn't change, labor didn't change—epidurals just weren't as easy to get.

Does this mean that women are suffering because they can't get epidurals, or that women at this hospital have lost some important choices in childbirth? Generally, when epidurals are less available, the nursing staff offer a wider array of methods for coping with labor pain. Women in hospitals where epidurals are readily available sometimes complain that they feel "pushed into having one." This demonstrates, perhaps, the challenges hospitals face in meeting the needs of all laboring women—from the mother who wants an epidural as early as possible to the mother who wants no interventions.

Most of the research about epidurals has compared one anesthetic with another. Considering how frequently epidural is used, it is staggering that there are virtually no data that explore the possible effects of epidural on either mother or baby in the long term. Studies that show the increased incidence of Caesarean section are quite recent, and there have been no good studies to explore if delaying epidural anesthetic until labor is well established would decrease the risk of vacuum or forceps delivery or Caesarean section.

Spinal Anesthesia

Spinal anesthesia is similar to epidural in that an intravenous is started first, and local anesthetic is put in through a needle in the back. The difference is that with a spinal anesthetic a much smaller needle is used and the dura (the lining around the spinal cord) is deliberately punctured so that the local anesthetic can be put right into the cerebrospinal fluid.

Spinal anesthetic gives extremely good pain relief for Caesarean section and for forceps deliveries, often better than can be achieved with an epidural. No catheter is left in place with spinal anesthesia, so pain control is not as prolonged or as controllable as epidural.

Complications of spinal anesthesia are similar to those for epidural. The drop in blood pressure after it is administered is even more frequent and severe than with epidural anesthetic, and pre-treatment with large volumes of intravenous fluid is typical.

About 1 percent of women get a "spinal headache," which lasts for three to five days. Mothers have been advised to lie flat, or have been given lots of fluid to prevent this, but these techniques have proven unsuccessful. In recent years, the incidence of spinal headache has been decreased by the use of extremely fine needles to do the spinal. If spinal headache occurs, a treatment called a "blood patch," in which a very small amount of the mother's blood is injected into the epidural space at the site of the puncture, is usually successful.

Narcotics can be injected into the cerebrospinal fluid as well as local anesthetic, and can give pain relief for up to 12 hours after a Caesarean section. There is recent interest in this method of pain control during the first stage of labor.

General Anesthesia

General anesthesia (going right to sleep) was used for years as pain relief for vaginal deliveries. This practice was discontinued for several reasons. There was a high risk of the baby being sleepy and not breathing properly after birth because the anesthetic crosses the placenta easily and quickly. There was a small risk of the mother vomiting while asleep and breathing the vomit into her lungs, causing aspiration pneumonia. Even though this was rare, it was an extremely serious complication.

Most importantly, epidural anesthesia was developed. The epidural was immediately much more popular with women, can be used for labor pain as well as delivery and eliminates the risk of aspiration pneumonia.

General anesthesia is still sometimes used for Caesarean sections, especially when a speedy delivery is critical, because a woman can be put to sleep faster than she can be given a spinal or epidural, without the same risk of the drop in blood pressure.

For planned Caesarean sections, where the woman is not in labor and has not eaten or drunk for the prescribed amount of time, general anesthesia or epidural or spinal anesthetic are all very safe choices. The decision may be offered to the woman, or the anesthetist or surgeon may have a preference.

The Evidence About . . .
PAIN IN LABOR

Few of the many drug-free approaches to easing labor pain provide dramatic pain relief, but many mothers find that they help them to cope with the pain they are experiencing.

Narcotics reduce pain in labor, but their usefulness is limited by their side-effects, particularly their effect on the baby's breathing.

Inhaling nitrous oxide is moderately effective in relieving pain, but can be difficult to use and may make the mother dizzy and nauseated.

Epidurals provide more effective pain relief than any other method, but substantially increase the risk of forceps or vacuum delivery and slightly increase the risk of Caesarean section. They also make the first stage of labor longer. Epidural anesthesia seems to be safe for the baby, but considering the frequency of use, there is remarkably little research on its effects on either mother or baby.

21

Labor and Its Variations: False Labor, Long Labor, Precipitate Labor

The day after her "due date" Cindy and her husband Rob were watching TV when she began to feel a cramping sensation in her abdomen. "It hurt," she said. "It wasn't like a menstrual cramp." When Rob put his hand on her belly, he could feel it getting tight, so he began to write down the times. After an hour, he noted that the contractions were pretty regular and about 10 minutes apart. They waited another hour, still recording the times, and decided to go to the hospital.

Cindy was very disappointed when the nurse who examined her found that her cervix was still firm and not dilated at all. The hospital staff suggested she go home and wait until the contractions got stronger and closer together. Within an hour after getting home, the contractions stopped. Her doctor explained, at her next prenatal visit, that she'd simply had a bout of false labor. Two weeks later, her water broke and her baby was born after an easy seven-hour labor.

Diane was 10 days past her "due date" with her third child when she woke up feeling "crampy—like having menstrual cramps." Her previous two births had involved a lot of back labor, so she didn't at first identify the cramps in her lower abdomen as contractions. "I thought maybe I had a bladder infection or something," she says. "Because I didn't feel anything in my back this time, I didn't think it could be labor."

The cramps continued throughout the day. "I had lots of things to do, but every now and then I'd have to sit down and catch my breath," says Diane. "Finally, I decided to call my doctor because I was concerned. It didn't really feel like my usual labor, but it wasn't going away." Her doctor told Diane to come to the hospital to be examined, and found she was well along in labor—7 cm (2.8 in) dilated. Diane's baby boy was born two hours later.

When Esther was expecting her third child, she had three episodes of false labor before the real thing arrived. "You'd think I'd know, after two previous babies," she says. Each time she called her midwife and had her support people gathered at her home, only to have the contractions fade away. "It was very embarrassing," she confesses.

When she woke up a few nights later with strong contractions, she decided to wait until she was absolutely certain it was "the real thing" before making any calls. By the time she was sure enough to wake up her husband Brian, labor was so strong she could barely talk and he had to make the calls to the others. When the midwife and Esther's friends arrived, the baby was already born. "Brian did a wonderful job catching the baby," Esther says, "but he did say I have to wake him up sooner next time."

As these stories demonstrate, it isn't easy to determine whether labor has really begun. Sometimes there will be strong contractions, but no apparent change in the cervix. Occasionally, the contractions will seem irregular or mild and yet the cervix is dilating quickly.

Other signs of labor are also unreliable. The membranes containing the amniotic fluid may break before labor starts or in early labor, but sometimes they don't break until the baby is actually being born. The mucus plug, which is in the center of the cervix, often comes away in early labor. The mother usually sees this as blood-tinged mucus on her underwear or in the toilet after she goes to the bathroom. Sometimes, though, pink-tinged mucus will be seen several days before labor starts.

Contractions may be regular and strong from the beginning, or they may take several hours to settle into a clear pattern. Sometimes the contractions stay quite far apart all through labor; in other cases they quickly become very close together, with little chance for a break or rest in between.

Because of these wide variations, women are often puzzled about when they should either go to the hospital or call the midwife if they are giving birth at home. Deciding when to go to the hospital can be important, because research has found that women who go to the hospital early in labor are more likely to be diagnosed with "abnormal labor," to receive more interventions and to have a Caesarean section than women who arrive at the hospital further along in labor.

So when should you go to the hospital (or call your midwife)? Your own feelings are the best guide. Would you really like to have your midwife with you to provide some reassurance and let you know what's happening? Are you feeling anxious about being at home and wanting to get into the hospital, or does the labor feel manageable at this point? Is the weather bad, so that it's best to leave extra travel time?

Are you worried because it's a long drive to the hospital? For women who have a long trip, deciding when to go is difficult. Perhaps you can go to the home of a friend who lives near the hospital, or stop in a park or the hospital grounds to walk for a while. (Of course, if it turns out to be false labor, you might end up going home again.)

How Labor Progresses

Labor progresses in two ways. First the cervix (which is like a thick, small donut with a tiny hole in the middle before labor starts) must thin out or *efface*. Then the cervix must open up or *dilate*. The contractions of labor move it from completely closed (0 cm or in dilated) to completely open (10 cm or 4 in dilated)—at this point the baby's head can come through the cervix and into the vagina to be born.

To check on the progress of your labor, the doctor, midwife or nurse will insert one hand into your vagina to feel the cervix and estimate how much it has opened. No studies have been done to see how precise these examinations are, but often different caregivers examining the same woman will give different numbers—

The first stage of labor: Before the onset of labor, the cervix is like a thick donut with a very small hole in the middle (top left). As labor progresses, the cervix first thins (top right), then opens (bottom left) to allow the baby to pass out of the uterus and into the vagina (bottom right).

a difference that could be important if there are concerns about how labor is progressing.

Early or latent labor is the time from the first contraction to the point where the cervix is 4 cm (1.6 in) dilated and 80 percent effaced. How long does this take? Some women have contractions for several days, or even weeks, and the cervix changes very slowly during this stage. Other women are not even aware of it—when they first notice contractions, they are already 4 or 5 cm (1.6 or 2 in) dilated. It can be very discouraging to the mother who has felt strong contractions for 12 hours or more to learn that she is only 2 cm (0.8 in) dilated and not even in active labor.

Long Latent Labor

What does it mean if this latent labor stage is longer than average? The studies tend to contradict themselves. Some see no higher complication rate with a long latent stage; others find that if it takes the mother a long time to dilate to 4 cm (1.6 in) she is more likely to have a forceps delivery or a Caesarean section. It's possible that the increased numbers of forceps or Caesarean births were caused by attempts to speed up the labor, rather than by the slow labor itself—the research doesn't make this clear.

Claire's labor with her second child started on a Friday evening. "I called my doula and she came over right away. The contractions were pretty solid ones, and I was glad to have both her and Glenn to help me get through them. We labored all night and then Saturday morning I had some bloody show, so we went to the hospital."

To Claire's disappointment, the nurse who examined her found that she was only about 1 cm (0.4 in) dilated. "I couldn't believe it. I'd been in labor something like 11 hours by then." Her doula reminded her that she was about 50 percent effaced, so the contractions

were working. They went back home and tried to rest.

Labor continued, though, and nobody got much rest. By Saturday night Claire was sure she must be further along, but another visit to the hospital found she was only 2 cm (0.8 in) dilated. This time she decided to stay, and wandered the hospital corridors with Glenn and the doula. It wasn't until very late Sunday night that she reached 4 cm (1.6 in) dilation, and then her labor got going; Claire's baby boy was born at 6 a.m. on Monday morning. "And then," she says, "I fell asleep."

Labor does not proceed at an even speed from beginning to end. In early labor, it may take several hours of contractions to dilate the cervix 1 cm (0.4 in), while at the end of labor the cervix may dilate 3 cm (1.2 in) in a few contractions.

A long latent phase of labor, and a longer labor overall, are more common when a first baby is being born. Usually subsequent labors are shorter—but not always.

Prolonged Labor

Measuring the rate of dilation of the cervix is only useful once the mother is in active labor. Once active labor is established, a rate of dilation of 0.5 to 1 cm (0.2 to 0.4 in) per hour is considered average. Sometimes doctors are concerned when labor is moving more slowly than average—if, for example, a mother who is 5 cm (2 in) dilated takes three hours to get to 6 cm (2.4 in). However, many women with slower-than-average rates of dilation have normal births.

Other factors should also be looked at before labor is considered to be progressing too slowly and in need of being "speeded up." Is the baby doing well, or showing signs of distress? Is the mother comfortable, walking around and coping with the contractions, or is she exhausted and overwhelmed? If mother and baby are both handling the slow labor well, there is probably little need for concern or intervention.

Maria's contractions were about six or seven minutes apart and it had taken her nearly 20 hours to get to 7 cm (2.8 in) dilation. If she sat down or lay down, her contractions would slow down to 10 or 12 minutes apart, so she kept walking, even though she was feeling tired. Periodic checks on the baby's heartbeat showed that he was doing well, and labor simply continued slowly but steadily. Four hours later, Maria's baby was born with the help of a vacuum extractor.

Women often find that their contractions slow down or stop temporarily when they arrive at the hospital. For most of us, a hospital is a fairly stressful environment, and stress significantly affects labor. Other sources of stress may also prolong labor—such as worrying about child care for your older children. Walking around has been clearly shown to speed up labor, and having a support person of your choosing present can also contribute to a shorter labor.

When active labor is going slowly, it may be labeled *failure to progress* or *dystocia*. Attempts to speed up the labor are called *augmenting* labor.

One common treatment is to rupture the membranes (called amniotomy). The doctor uses an instrument like a crochet hook to break the membranes open; the mother will not feel any pain, only the sudden gush of warm fluid. When this is done routinely fairly early in labor, it can shorten the time until the baby is born by one or two hours. No adverse effects have been demonstrated in research studies. However, there are concerns that if the labor turns out to be false—in other words, if contractions stop—the ruptured membranes may increase the risk of infection. For that reason, this should only be used when labor is clearly

underway. Unfortunately, when amniotomy is specifically used to speed up labors that are progressing slowly, it is less effective.

Another very common way to augment the labor is to give a synthetic form of the hormone oxytocin intravenously. This is usually done if spontaneous or artificial rupture of the membranes has not made the labor speed up.

Is oxytocin effective to speed up labor? Studies have found that women given oxytocin will dilate more quickly when compared with women who are kept in bed during labor, but more slowly than those who walk around during labor. There did not seem to be increased complications or problems for the babies when oxytocin was given.

However, most of the mothers who had been given oxytocin in the hopes of speeding up labor said it made their contractions more painful and they found the treatment unpleasant. Only a small percentage of the mothers who walked during labor said they found the contractions more painful when they walked.

In general, walking around is as effective as giving oxytocin in labor, and more comfortable for the mother. If the mother is feeling too tired to walk, or she is unable to walk because of pain-killing drugs or epidural, however, oxytocin is helpful in augmenting labor and making it go faster. Since women vary in how sensitive they are to oxytocin, the best method is to give small doses initially, increasing the amount every 30 minutes while watching the contractions carefully.

Fast Labor

What about labor that goes too fast? A *precipitate labor*—one that is very intense and quick—sounds ideal to many pregnant women, but mothers who have experienced them are less enthusiastic. The intensity of the contractions can be overwhelming, and often the mother is frightened about giving birth unexpectedly

Labor that Doesn't Progress: Marina's Story

Some labors don't progress to the normal, vaginal birth of a baby, no matter how patient the mother or how skilled the caregiver. Marina and John vividly remember their two long and unproductive labors.

John says, "With our first baby, Marina finally started to have contractions at six o'clock on Saturday morning–two weeks after her due date. The contractions seemed to come and go. Some were really hard and painful, some just made her stop walking for a minute. That night, the midwife came to check Marina. Even though she'd been having contractions all day, her cervix hadn't dilated at all.

"We tried to get some sleep, but Marina was too uncomfortable. On Sunday we tried everything we could think of to make the contractions stronger and closer. We walked for miles. We danced. We sang that Bob Dylan song: "Ooowee, ride me high, tomorrow's the day my baby's gonna come." But the baby didn't come. By Sunday night, we were both exhausted. The midwife checked again and Marina was just 2 cm (0.8 in) dilated. We decided to go to the hospital."

The doctor suggested breaking Marina's water, and that brought on stronger and more painful contractions. By Monday morning, Marina was finding the pain just about unbearable. But after all those contractions, she'd only dilated one more centimeter (0.4 in).

John continues: "Marina decided to have an epidural for the pain, and as soon as it took effect she fell asleep. Four hours later, though, she still hadn't dilated any more. The decision was easy–this baby would be born by Caesarean section. I was so exhausted that the masks and lights in the operating room were almost surreal. Jesse cried right away as soon as he was lifted out of Marina's belly."

Two years later, John and Marina conceived a second child. Marina says, "I still wanted to have a vaginal labor and birth. I talked to my doctor a lot, and decided not to think too much about the first Caesarean, but just to go into labor and see what happened."

Once again, Marina went past her due date. "My contractions were fairly regular and got quite strong after a few hours. Then my water broke, and they got really painful and close together. We went to the hospital, and the nurse was sure I'd be delivering soon because I was in such hard labor. But when my doctor examined me, I was hardly dilated at all."

Marina walked around for the next eight hours, groaning through intense contractions, but when her doctor examined her, she was only 2 cm (0.8 in) dilated. "I could see that this was going the same way as Jesse's birth, and we decided–after 22 hours of labor–to have another Caesarean."

Marina says, "I'm still disappointed that I couldn't give birth vaginally. My doctor couldn't tell me why it happened this way–she says we just don't know why some cervixes don't dilate. I'm not happy that I had Caesareans, but I am glad they were available when I needed them."

without the opportunity to get to the hospital. Also, there is a higher risk of heavy bleeding after the baby is born.

Colleen's labor started very abruptly late on a Saturday night. "The contractions just hit me all of a sudden, and they were really strong and close together. I knew the baby was going to come soon, so I told my husband we'd better get moving."

They drove to the hospital, and Colleen felt the contractions getting even stronger. "The hospital's only about 15 minutes from our house, but it seemed like the longest drive I ever did." They parked the car, and as they began to walk towards the hospital entrance, Colleen's water broke.

"That did it," she says. "I knew the baby was coming *now*. All I could think was that I didn't want to have the baby on the pavement, so I made my way to the grass, pulled my shorts off, and lay down on the grass just in time for the baby to come out."

As Colleen lay on the grass, holding her newborn daughter, her husband ran into the hospital. He shouted that his wife had just had a baby "on the grass" and rushed back out to be with her. Unfortunately, he ran back out again so quickly that the nurses couldn't see which way he had gone in the dark. Several nurses fanned out and began searching the area around the hospital. It wasn't long before they discovered Colleen and her newborn, and the

---

The Evidence About...
LABOR AND ITS VARIATIONS

The variations in labor can be pretty dramatic—from very slow to very fast—and yet all fall within the range of "normal." It's these variations that make it hard to plan for labor and birth, because each experience is unique.

Artificial rupture of the membranes in early labor makes the labor shorter by an average of one to two hours, without causing any other complications. It is, however, less effective when used in slowly progressing labors.

If labor is progressing slowly, walking is as effective as oxytocin to speed it up and more comfortable for the mother. If walking is impossible because of fatigue or drugs, oxytocin is an effective way of augmenting labor.

---

new family was ushered into the hospital to get cleaned up.

Colleen can laugh about it now. "I know what story we'll be telling at her wedding," she says. But at the time it was pretty frightening, and Colleen worried that the baby would be injured by the rapid birth.

22

Here Comes the Baby! The Second (Pushing) Stage

"I have to push."

For many women, the point at which they first feel the baby moving down and their bodies beginning to push the baby out is one of the most exciting moments of labor. Those pushing sensations tell them that the birth of the baby is close and labor is almost over. It can also be a relief to be actively involved, after hours of just trying to cope with contractions.

Bonnie remembers: "My labor had been a lot more painful than I had expected. I had only been in labor five hours and I was groaning and finding it pretty unbearable. I remember saying to my husband, 'I can't do this any more.' He was struggling to find something supportive and comforting to say—actually he looked scared to death every time I groaned—when all of a sudden my water broke and my body pushed.

"I yelled, 'I'm pushing!' He raced out of the room to get the nurse—I think he thought the baby was going to fall right out on the floor. From then on, the labor was great. The pushing urge was absolutely overwhelming during the contractions—I can't imagine any woman asking if it's time to push. The pushing contractions were really intense, but nothing as painful as the contractions had been up to then.

"In no time at all—my husband says it was about half an hour—I could feel the baby sort of bulging in my vagina. I can't remember if the nurse or my doctor tried to tell me when to push—it wouldn't have mattered what they said, my body just did it. It felt amazing when the baby slid out—it just burned, it really didn't hurt at all."

Maria's memory of her baby's birth is very different, but equally happy: "I'd had an epidural when I was 8 cm (3.2 in), and promptly went to sleep. I woke up when the nurse came in to do a routine check. She said that I was fully dilated and that the baby's head was right at the opening of the vagina! I couldn't feel a thing—not just the pain was gone, I had no sensation at all.

"The nurse and doctor tried to get me to push when they told me I had a contraction, but all I could do was laugh, I was so excited.

They had a mirror so I could see the top of the baby's head—it was unbelievable. The doctor put a plastic thing on Chantelle's head and pulled a bit and out she came, all pink and beautiful. It was all so wonderful because there wasn't a bit of pain—I completely enjoyed the baby's birth."

The second stage of labor begins when the cervix is fully dilated, and ends with the birth of the baby. How will you feel when the second stage begins? The desire to push doesn't always coincide with the moment the cervix finishes dilating. Some mothers feel strong pushing urges before full dilation, and others don't feel pushing urges for some time after the cervix is fully dilated. Sometimes labor seems to slow down at this point, with contractions coming further apart; other women find that contractions are closer together. With epidural anesthetic, some mothers never feel any pushing urge at all.

There is also a difference between the sensation of "feeling like pushing," which women experience during a contraction, and the actual involuntary "push" that the abdominal muscles give as the baby's head comes down into the pelvis.

Most of the advice you may be given about what to do during the second stage is based on "clinical experience" (meaning the way your physician has always done it) and has not been researched. Nearly all the research that has been done has involved very small studies using very few women.

Should Women Be Told How to Push?

Women who are given no directions at all during the pushing stage react to it in very similar ways. Even if they report "feeling like pushing," they seldom make themselves push on purpose. Once the urge to push becomes involuntary, they usually make three to five relatively brief pushes (four to six seconds each) during each contraction. There is usually little holding of the breath—air is released, often with a grunt, during each push.

This is quite different from the way women are often instructed to push. A nurse or other birth attendant may tell you to take a big breath in, hold your breath and then to push down for a sustained period of time, from 10 to 30 seconds. You might practice this pushing during prenatal classes. Women are often told to push this way as soon as they are fully dilated, whether they have any spontaneous urge to push or not.

The coached, holding-your-breath type of pushing results in a slightly shorter second stage, but otherwise has no benefits for mother or baby. Spontaneous (mother-directed) pushing results in better fetal heart rate patterns, higher Apgar scores at birth and higher pH in the umbilical cord blood (all indicative of better fetal well-being).

Interestingly, women with epidural anesthetic are often encouraged to bear down forcefully as soon as full dilation is diagnosed by a vaginal examination (because of the anesthetic they often do not feel any pushing urge). If instead you wait until the baby's head appears in the vagina to start pushing, studies show that you are less likely to need forceps to turn the baby's head from a posterior position.

Positions for Pushing

Standing, kneeling or squatting to give birth is common in most cultures. It has not been common in ours—in hospitals, women have almost universally been encouraged to lie on their backs to deliver, often with their legs up in leg rests or stirrups.

Several small studies have compared being upright for birth with lying down. "Lying down" has meant either the mother lying on her back or on her side. "Upright" has meant being propped up by a backrest or wedge on a bed, or using a specially designed birthing chair. Squatting (with or without support from a low birthing stool) or kneeling has not been researched at all.

Being upright shortens the length of the second stage. Mothers prefer being upright because they feel less pain and less backache, and a majority of the women said they wanted to use the same upright position for their next birth. Abnormal fetal heart rate patterns and low umbilical cord pH (both signs of fetal distress) were slightly less likely with the upright position.

Women who give birth lying on their sides also have infants with better heart rate patterns and better umbilical cord pH than those who deliver lying on their backs. It seems that both the upright and the side-lying positions avoid the compression of the blood vessels by the uterus that is caused by lying on the back.

Studies did not find any differences in the rate of tears in the vagina depending on pushing position. Studies also have not shown any change in the rates of vacuum, forceps or Caesarean section between upright posture and lying down for the second stage. However, the studies have been very small, and have included women in the "upright" group who simply had a support or backrest under their head and shoulders while they were on their back in bed with their legs in stirrups.

"Birthing chairs" are just that—a chair in which the woman sits, usually leaning back, to give birth. The use of birthing chairs leads to a higher risk of swollen perineum, hemorrhoids and postpartum hemorrhage if the mother sits in the chair for extended periods of time. This seems to be related to the construction of the chair itself, which puts pressure on the thighs and reduces blood flow back from the legs.

Giving birth while lying on your back has not been found to have any benefits to you or your baby.

Vaginal Tears

Delivery of the baby can tear the tissue around the opening of the vagina (the perineum). This probably happens in about 50 percent of births. (We don't really know how many women would tear if they were left alone, because so many are given episiotomies, a cut made by the doctor in the tissue between the opening of the vagina and the anus, at the time of birth.)

Clearly, in the days before sutures (stitches) were invented, women had babies, got tears and most of them healed fine by themselves (although it's also certain that some of the tears didn't heal well and caused the mother a lot of trouble).

The current assumption is that all tears, except for the tiniest, should be sutured. There is no research to support this. One study looked at episiotomies that had been repaired with sutures but "broke down." One group was left to heal by themselves; the other group was resutured. The group who were resutured healed faster and had fewer complications. This study would support the already accepted procedure of suturing all *significant* tears. It's not clear, though, that this should apply to smaller tears.

Preventing Tears

There is no evidence about the best method of preventing the perineum from tearing during delivery. Many techniques have been suggested:

- Leaving the perineum strictly alone.
- "Guarding" the perineum by the caregiver pressing her fingers against it, combined with gentle pressure on the baby's head to prevent rapid delivery.
- Massaging the perineum with warm oil (either just at birth or for several weeks before the baby is born).
- Applying hot compresses to the perineum to help the tissues stretch.
- Avoiding coached pushing, except at the moment of birth. Then the caregiver encourages the mother to pant or blow steadily out as the baby's head begins to be born. Her uterus will continue to contract and push the baby out but will do so slowly, giving the skin the maximum amount of time to stretch. (This kind of slow birth is sometimes hard to achieve, as some women can't stop pushing.)

None of these methods—all of which have passionate advocates—have been researched to see if they are effective in preventing tears to the vagina. They may be effective, but the research has never been done. This is an example of research that would be of great interest to women.

Some of these techniques at least make the mother feel more comfortable at the time. Marjory remembers: "The hot compresses on my vagina felt so good—they absolutely took away all the pain from pushing. I wouldn't let the midwife stop doing them for one second. I tore just a little when the baby came out—I don't know if the compresses kept it from being any worse, but they sure felt good."

What feels great to one mother may distress another. Elyse says, "Before I had Danny, I had discussed with my doctor not having an episiotomy. She said she massages the perineum with warm oil, and it sounded great. But when I was actually pushing and she started to rub the oil onto me, I couldn't stand it. I actually yelled at her to stop; I was so hypersensitive even that gentle touch felt painful."

Episiotomy

Gary still vividly remembers seeing his wife Lisa being given an episiotomy. After 19 hours of labor, she was finally fully dilated and beginning to push out her baby. She was tired and the doctor and nurse urged her to push harder. Gary held up one of her legs, braced against his shoulder, while the nurse held the other leg. Then the doctor reached over to the green cloth laid out on a metal table and picked up a pair of scissors.

"I'd gotten through labor fine," Gary says, "but when I saw the doctor make that cut, I almost passed out."

Lisa's response was less dramatic. "I think I was feeling so much pain and pressure at that point that I didn't really notice what the doctor was doing. But I noticed it afterwards."

During the birth of Lisa's daughter, the episiotomy tore even further. The doctor stitched up both the episiotomy and the tearing. "It took forever," Lisa recalls, and she felt uncomfortable for several months afterwards. When she became pregnant again, Lisa sought out a new doctor who supported her desire to avoid another episiotomy. During her second birth she had only a small tear requiring a few stitches, which was pain-free in about a week.

An episiotomy is a cut made in the perineum to enlarge the opening before the baby's head comes through. Sometimes the cut is done straight down from the bottom of the vagina, and other times it is done at an angle. While episiotomies are less commonly done than in the past, between 50 and 90 percent of women in North America have an episiotomy at the birth of their first child. The rates vary dramatically among physicians. Some doctors will try to avoid an episiotomy with a second or later birth, even if they usually do one for a first baby.

The stated reasons why episiotomies are routinely performed are not supported by the research that has been done.

To study the potential benefits and disadvantages of episiotomies, women were divided into two groups. In one group, episiotomies were done "liberally," meaning that most women received them. In this group, however, there were still some women who delivered their babies so quickly the doctor didn't have time to do the episiotomy. The other group was "restricted" in terms of episiotomy, meaning that they were done very seldom, and only when there was a clear need (such as a difficult forceps delivery or a baby in distress).

When the groups were compared, it was clear that there were no benefits to the liberal use of episiotomy.

- Episiotomies to shorten the pushing stage of labor do not prevent damage to the baby's head and brain. Babies born without episiotomy need no more resuscitation or intensive care than babies born with episiotomy.
- Episiotomy does not protect the mother from "worse tearing." Tearing that damages the muscles around the mother's anus and rectum occurs significantly *more* often—not less—when a midline episiotomy is done than when a spontaneous tear happens during the delivery.
- The number of women who have stress incontinence three years after delivery is the same whether they had an episiotomy or not. (Stress incontinence is a fairly common problem in women—when they cough or sneeze or laugh hard, particularly if their bladder is full, they leak some urine.)

Episiotomy does not prevent damage to the bladder muscles and other muscles of the pelvic floor.

- There is no evidence that episiotomies heal better than tears. Women who had episiotomies and women who didn't had the same amount of pain at 10 days and at three months postpartum. However, the women who did not have episiotomies started to have sex again sooner than the women who did.

Risks of Episiotomy

Episiotomy can cause excessive blood loss from the wound edges, particularly if the cut is made well before the delivery of the baby. It can also cause infection and abscess formation, injury to the muscles of the anus and rectum and a hole (called a fistula) between the rectum and the vagina.

When Is Episiotomy Useful?

There are times when an episiotomy may be helpful:

- If the baby coming through the vagina is in distress and needs to be born quickly, an episiotomy may help speed up the birth.
- If forceps or a vacuum extractor is needed to help the baby emerge, an episiotomy may provide extra room for inserting the instrument to pull the baby out, and in the case of a difficult birth also allows more room for the baby.
- For a breech birth, the smaller body and legs come out first and then the larger head and shoulders have to be born quickly so that the baby can start to breathe. The smaller parts coming first have not stretched the perineum very much, so the head can be a tight fit. Doing an episiotomy when the buttocks reach the perineum may offer some protection to the baby's head and

avoid a difficult delivery. This has not been researched, but it is done almost routinely.

Roxanne remembers her episiotomy vividly: "My doctor and I were in agreement that episiotomies were unnecessary. My labor had gone great, I was pushing, the pain wasn't too bad. The nurse had set up a mirror so I could see my baby's head in the vagina with each contraction. The baby's heart rate had been fine—then after one contraction it was really slow. We could all hear it just going . . . thud . . . thud . . . thud, when before it had been quick.

"My doctor said that sometimes the baby's head gets squeezed at this stage and it doesn't necessarily mean the baby is in distress. I rolled over onto my side and the nurse gave me some oxygen to breathe.

"The baby's heart rate speeded up a little with the next couple of contractions, but it was still a lot slower than it had been. The doctor said she couldn't tell for sure whether the baby was in distress, and the quickest way to get the baby born would be to do an episiotomy. I told her to go ahead—I was pretty worried—so she put in some freezing and did an episiotomy with the next contraction.

"The baby's head came out; the cord was around her neck and the doctor had to cut the cord before her shoulders came out. The baby was a bit quiet for a minute, and the doctor rubbed her and gave her some oxygen to breathe. Then she started to cry and everything was fine."

Vacuum Extractors and Forceps

If the mother's efforts to push her baby out don't seem to be working, either forceps or the vacuum extractor can be used to help deliver the baby. The cervix must be fully dilated and the baby's head must be engaged. "Engaged"

Pain Relief for Episiotomy

Freezing with local anesthetic is needed for an episiotomy, unless the woman already has an epidural in place. The freezing can be injected directly into the skin of the perineum that is going to be cut. Another type of anesthetic for an episiotomy, which also gives some pain relief for a vacuum or low forceps delivery, is a pudendal block. Local anesthetic is injected through the sidewalls of the vagina into the pudendal nerves. This does not give the same complete pain relief given by an epidural, but it does make the whole vaginal area less sensitive.

means that the baby's head has moved down under the pubic bone into the pelvis, so that the widest part of the baby's head is in the pelvis. That's usually a good sign that the head will fit through the bones of the pelvis, and that the vacuum or forceps will just be helping to stretch the soft tissues of the perineum.

If the baby's head is *not* engaged, forceps or vacuum are usually not tried because of concerns that the baby simply isn't going to fit through the bony pelvis. If that is the case, pulling on it might damage the baby, without being able to deliver it, and a Caesarean section is probably safer for the baby.

Forceps

"I had been pushing for about two and a half hours," says Ann, remembering the birth of her first baby. "I didn't seem to be making any progress at all. My doctor explained that the baby was posterior—face-up—and that she'd like to use forceps to turn him."

Ann was feeling tired after a long labor and the time she had spent pushing. "I really felt like the baby wasn't moving at all, so we went for the forceps. I was very disappointed that I had to have an epidural at that point, after going through the whole labor without any drugs. And I had a big episiotomy, too. But a few minutes later, I had my baby in my arms."

Forceps, like the ones Ann's doctor used, are metal instruments that look roughly like salad tongs. They fit around the baby's head, and then the doctor pulls on them to deliver the baby. They can also be used to turn the baby's head from a posterior position (with the face looking up) to an anterior position (with the face looking down). In an anterior position, the baby's head usually fits through the pelvis better and will deliver more easily.

The safety of forceps for the baby depends completely on the physician's training, experience and judgment. Skill is needed to turn the baby's head gently without undue force. When pulling, the baby's head should move down somewhat with each pull—it takes good judgment to decide when a forceps delivery is going to use too much force and it is safer to do a Caesarean section instead.

Low forceps—a forceps delivery done when the baby's head is at the opening of the vagina—can usually be done with local anesthetic to freeze the opening of the vagina. Mid forceps—a forceps delivery done when the baby is higher in the birth canal, will usually mean the mother needs epidural anesthesia to handle the pain. Most forceps deliveries that involve rotations of the baby's head from the posterior or transverse position to the anterior position are mid forceps.

Vacuum Extractor

The vacuum extractor is a soft plastic cup about the size of an egg that is slipped into the vagina and pressed against the baby's head. It has tubing attached that is connected to a pump; the pump creates a vacuum between the cup and the baby's scalp. During contrac-

tions, the vacuum is increased and the physician pulls on the extractor to help with delivery. Between contractions, the vacuum is released so that it won't create a pressure sore on the baby's scalp.

The built-in safety of the vacuum extractor is the ease with which the cup "pops off" the baby's scalp. It is difficult to pull hard enough to harm the baby without the vacuum letting go.

The cup often produces a swollen area on the baby's scalp from the vacuum, which is harmless and usually disappears within 48 hours. At times, there can be bleeding into this swollen area, causing a bruise on the baby's head. This takes longer to heal, but causes the baby no lasting harm.

A vacuum extraction can usually be done with just a local anesthetic.

Deciding to Use Forceps or Vacuum Extractors

Marilyn had been fully dilated for about half an hour and was pushing each time the nurse reading the monitor told her a contraction was coming. Because she'd had an epidural, she didn't feel any pushing urge. When her doctor came in to observe, he told her that things were moving slowly.

"I can get this baby out now with a vacuum extractor," he said, "and you won't have to wait any longer to have him in your arms."

What are good reasons for using forceps or the vacuum? The most common ones given are:

Fetal Distress: If your baby is in distress during this pushing stage, forceps or vacuum can help deliver the baby. However, it isn't easy to diagnose fetal distress at this point. If the baby's heart rate is very slow and not speeding up between contractions, it is probably in distress.

But what about patterns that are less clear-cut? Often during the pushing stage a baby's heartbeat will slow down during contractions, then speed up again once the contraction ends. This seems to be normal and is probably caused by the squeezing of the baby's head as it pushes through the birth canal during contractions. However, if the umbilical cord is around the baby's neck, you will see the same pattern of changing heart rate: slow during contractions, faster in between. In the early stages, it's impossible to tell the difference between the normal changes in heart rate and the potentially dangerous cord around the baby's neck. (The baby with a tight cord around its neck will show more serious signs of distress as it moves farther down the birth canal.)

It also gets increasingly difficult to hear the baby's heartbeat as the pushing stage continues. You may notice the nurse or midwife placing the stethoscope on various parts of your belly as she tries to find a good place to listen. If you are moving around, trying to find a comfortable position for pushing, it can get even harder. If you are on your hands and knees, for example, or sitting backwards on the toilet, your caregiver may find it very challenging to listen to your baby.

Long Second Stage: No studies have been performed to determine how long it is safe for the mother to push, or at what point in time the use of vacuum or forceps should be considered. A very long second stage is statistically associated with stillbirths, postpartum hemorrhage, fever in the mother and seizures in the newborn. However, there is no evidence that the length of the second stage itself causes these complications.

The average length of the second stage for mothers having their first baby is about an hour, and for women having subsequent babies is about 30 minutes. That's just an average, though, and there are wide variations. Many doctors use as their definition of an abnormally long second stage two hours for a first birth,

and one hour for a second birth; after this they suggest the use of vacuum or forceps.

This arbitrary clock-watching is not supported by research. If the mother is not exhausted, the baby's condition is fine (as shown by normal heart rate) and the baby's head is continuing to move down through the birth canal, there is no reason to arbitrarily put a time limit on the second stage.

If you have had an epidural and have no pushing urge, it is reasonable to expect a longer second stage to allow the contractions to move the baby down to the opening of the vagina. Sometimes, the combination of epidural anesthesia and the reaching of full dilation drastically slows down the frequency of the contractions. In this case, oxytocin might make the contractions more frequent and allow you to give birth without using forceps or vacuum.

You can be involved in making this decision. If you are exhausted and in pain from a long labor and pushing stage, you may want to "get things over with" by having an epidural and forceps or vacuum to deliver the baby. If you are feeling fine and the baby is doing well, however, you can tell your doctor that you would like to continue.

Marilyn chose to wait. "Because of the epidural, I wasn't in any pain, and I knew I'd need an episiotomy if I had the vacuum extractor. It took another 45 minutes before Amy was born, but I only had a small tear, so I was glad we let her arrive at her own speed."

Are Forceps Deliveries Safe for the Baby?

There are really two different questions here. If the forceps have been used during a straightforward, normal labor and birth simply to shorten the second stage, we want to know if this is safer than a natural, vaginal birth. But if the forceps were used because the mother had

Forceps versus Vacuum?

The first decision to be made is whether either one of these interventions is appropriate. Would waiting a little longer, or trying a different position, be effective and safe?

If intervention is necessary, vacuum extractor tried first, followed by forceps if that fails, results in a lower Caesarean rate. However, the most important factor is probably the skill, judgment and experience of the doctor.

been pushing for several hours and the baby was not coming out, we should be asking if forceps are safer than a Caesarean section, because that would have been the alternative.

Forceps used in a straightforward birth do not seem to cause any harm to the baby.

Forceps deliveries can be just as safe as Caesarean sections in more difficult births, provided certain guidelines are followed. The cervix must be fully dilated and the baby's head must be well down in the mother's pelvis. In this situation, many doctors will try using forceps before suggesting the surgery. If the forceps don't work—if the doctor needs to use a lot of force, for example—the baby will be delivered promptly by Caesarean section instead.

Which Is Better, Forceps or Vacuum Extractor?

In North America, forceps have been used much more than the vacuum, while in Europe, the use of the vacuum is more common than forceps.

The vacuum extractor usually requires less pain-relieving medication for the mother. It is less likely to cause tears to the mother's vagina, and causes less pain after the birth. The vacuum extractor frequently causes swelling or bruising of the baby's scalp, while the forceps are more likely to cause cuts or bruises on the baby's face.

As far as getting the baby born quickly, the effectiveness of the vacuum extractor and forceps is about the same. It usually takes slightly longer, depending on the hospital, to arrange for an epidural for the mother in order to use forceps. The vacuum extractor is not successful as often as forceps in getting the baby out. However, if the vacuum extractor is tried first, followed by forceps if the vacuum doesn't work, the overall Caesarean section rate is lower.

Since the vacuum extractor causes fewer problems for the mother and requires less medication, it is usually the best first choice. However, your doctor's skill and experience with a technique is the best guarantee of safety, and will be an important factor in making the choice between vacuum and forceps.

In some hospitals, women are frequently encouraged to have the vacuum extractor used to speed up the births of their babies. Since the vacuum doesn't require an epidural, and is seen as safe for both mother and baby, it has become popular. There is no research to show that this routine use of the vacuum is beneficial, or that it is dangerous.

The Evidence About ...
PUSHING THE BABY OUT

There are many strongly held opinions about the pushing stage of labor, but not much research.

Babies are born in better condition when the mother is not coached on how to push, but when she pushes spontaneously. With this approach, the second stage is only a little longer than when pushing is coached.

Being upright during the second stage is more comfortable for most women, makes the second stage shorter and slightly improves the condition of the baby when born.

There are many theories, but no proof, of the best way (if there is a best way) to prevent tearing at delivery.

There is no evidence of *any* benefits from the liberal use of episiotomy. Using episiotomy to avoid a tear is counterproductive, as the risk of tearing is higher when an episiotomy is done.

Research has not established the maximum length of time for the pushing stage that is safe for mother and baby. Setting arbitrary time limits is probably not helpful.

If the baby is not born in a "reasonable" length of time, either vacuum extraction or forceps can be used as long as the cervix is fully dilated and the baby's head is engaged. Vacuum extraction is probably safer for mother and baby, but is not as successful as often as forceps.

23

The Third Stage of Labor: Delivery of the Placenta

Your baby's born and in your arms. It's over at last, and as you gaze into your baby's eyes you know it was worth it. Then, to your surprise, you feel another contraction...

Well, it's not quite over. Yes, the birth of the baby is what you've been waiting for. But your body has another task to take care of—expelling the no-longer-needed placenta from your uterus. This is called the third stage of labor, and it seems like an anticlimax. Who wants to think about the placenta with a brand-new baby to cuddle and admire?

However, your caregiver needs to be alert at this time because there are potential hazards. It's possible for you to bleed heavily at this point, and that can be serious. In fact, it happens in about 8 percent of births. If the placenta doesn't come out on its own, this is called a "retained placenta" and the doctor may have to remove it (you will usually have anesthesia if this is necessary). In very rare cases, the uterus can turn inside out and come out of the vagina with the placenta—a very dangerous situation.

The best approach to the third stage of labor will be one that interferes as little as possible with the body's own normal process of delivering the placenta, minimizes the risk of serious complications like hemorrhage and retained placenta and doesn't disturb the mother's enjoyment of her new baby.

How Is the Placenta Normally Expelled?
After the delivery of the baby, the uterus immediately contracts to a firm ball about the size of a cantaloupe. The placenta, however, stays the same size and separates from the uterine wall as the uterus contracts. The contracted uterus then pushes the detached placenta into the lower uterine segment and into the vagina.

You can often watch your uterus becoming firmer and rounder just above your pelvic bone as the placenta moves down. There is often a sudden gush of blood from the vagina as well. If you have not been given an epidural, and particularly if you are upright, you will probably feel a slight urge to push at this point, and the placenta will slide easily out of your vagina.

If you are lying down, or have been given anesthetic so that you don't feel any sensation from the placenta in your vagina, your caregiver may put one hand on your uterus to support it and ask you to push gently. Along with gentle traction (pulling) on the umbilical cord, this is usually enough to expel the placenta from the vagina.

Once the placenta is delivered, a nurse or midwife will massage your uterus to make sure it stays firm and contracted and to minimize the amount of bleeding. This can sometimes be quite painful, depending on how vigorously it is done.

Ingrid says, "I hardly noticed the placenta coming out, because I was so absorbed by Jackson. I have vague memories of the doctor telling me to push and somebody showing me what looked like a big hunk of liver in a bowl. Then the nurse kind of grabbed at my belly and started to massage me—and I noticed that! When she saw my reaction, though, she realized she was doing it too hard, and tried to be a bit more gentle."

Hemorrhage after the Baby Is Born

About 8 percent of women will bleed heavily after delivery of their baby or the placenta—heavily enough to make their blood pressure fall, feel faint and need transfusion with intravenous fluid and/or blood. This is called postpartum hemorrhage, and it is slightly more likely in women who:

- have an overstretched uterus, because of a very large baby, twins or triplets, or a large amount of amniotic fluid;
- have very long or very short labors;

The Placenta

Many mothers want to see the placenta once it has been delivered. It is often larger than parents expect, and looks like a generous slab of liver. One side is raw-looking; this is the part that was attached to the uterus. The other side is smooth and shiny and the umbilical cord emerges from the middle of it. This side faced the baby before birth.

Your midwife or doctor will carefully examine the placenta to see that it has come away in one piece. If a piece is left behind in the uterus, it can lead to heavy bleeding.

- have had several previous births;
- have had a postpartum hemorrhage with a previous birth.

If this bleeding happens before the placenta is out, the placenta needs to be delivered as quickly as possible. If the placenta has separated from the uterus and is just sitting in the lower uterine segment or in the vagina, your doctor will probably pull on the umbilical cord to get it out. You will also be given oxytocin or ergometrine, drugs that make the uterus contract. Ergometrine is more likely than oxytocin to cause nausea, vomiting, headache and temporary elevation of blood pressure.

If the placenta has not separated from the uterus and the mother is bleeding heavily, the doctor may need to manually remove the placenta by putting his or her hand inside the uterus and prying the placenta away. If you have had an epidural, the doctor will be able to do this right away; if not, you will be given a general anesthetic. You also will be given oxytocin by intravenous. Some research has suggested that injecting oxytocin into the umbilical cord can help the placenta to separate and reduce the need to remove the placenta manually.

Priya had an eight-hour labor without any pain medication. "It was very straightforward—the nurses were joking that I'd be great for one of those childbirth videos. I was so thrilled when Sanjay was born, but then the placenta didn't come out. The doctor waited a while, tried massaging my belly, everything we could think of. Then I felt this gush of blood, and the doctor got concerned." Priya was quickly moved to another room and given a general anesthetic while the placenta was removed. "I felt so groggy when I woke up, but I knew it was necessary. I have to admit it was pretty disappointing to have that happen when the labor and birth went so well, but there are some things you just can't predict."

Prevention of Postpartum Hemorrhage

Prevention is better than treatment. Large studies have been done on giving either oxytocin or ergometrine routinely to women right after birth, and both made a significant difference in the amount of bleeding. These trials have shown *a reduction of about 60 percent in incidence of postpartum hemorrhage in women given oxytocin or ergometrine routinely after delivery of the baby.* Since oxytocin has fewer side-effects, it is preferred.

Clamping the Umbilical Cord

Should the umbilical cord be clamped later or earlier?

The usual practice in North America has been to clamp and cut the umbilical cord as soon as the baby is born. However, some have suggested that waiting for a period of time after the baby is born to clamp the cord is better because it allows as much blood as possible to

Should Dad Cut the Cord?

Some fathers see cutting the umbilical cord as a symbolic moment, and are eager to take part; others find they are too emotionally caught up in the birth to take on this role. If you are interested, ask your caregiver—you may also need to remind him or her at the time of the birth.

Your doctor or midwife will put clamps on the cord in two places, and you will be handed a pair of scissors to cut through the cord between the two clamps. It is slippery and a bit tough, like a garden hose. Neither mother nor baby will feel anything, and because of the clamps on either side, there will be almost no blood.

flow into the baby. Different researchers have adopted different definitions of "late" clamping—waiting for 30 seconds after delivery, or until the cord has stopped pulsing completely, or until after the placenta is delivered. The amount of extra blood the baby gets when the cord is clamped later also depends on positioning—the baby should be level with or slightly below the level of the vaginal opening for the blood to flow downhill.

When the cord is cut right after the baby is born, the baby will have lower blood volume and lower levels of iron. These differences generally disappear by the time the baby is six months old. However, the difference may be significant for premature babies—the cord is often clamped early to facilitate their resuscitation, but they might benefit from the extra blood.

The time of cord clamping does not seem to have anything to do with the risk of hemorrhage. Early cord clamping does reduce the length of time until the placenta delivers. If you would prefer to have the clamping of the cord delayed so that your baby gets the extra blood, be sure to discuss this with your doctor.

Controlled Traction on the Cord to Deliver the Placenta

At many births, the doctor pulls on the umbilical cord to remove the placenta from the vagina. "Controlled" cord traction is such a subjective thing that it is difficult to study meaningfully—there is no way to assess just how hard someone is pulling!

In one study, about 3 percent of the cords broke while traction was being used. If the cord breaks, sometimes the placenta will still deliver spontaneously, but sometimes it means that the placenta has not separated from the uterus, and a manual removal will be required.

How Soon Should the Placenta Be Delivered?

Most placentas will deliver within five to ten minutes of the delivery of the baby.

If there is no unusual bleeding, it is reasonable to wait an hour for spontaneous separation and delivery of the placenta rather than moving immediately to manual removal. Waiting an hour rather than half an hour has greatly reduced the number of manual removals required.

Stella's son, Neil, was born at home, but the placenta was slow in coming. "The midwives helped me to squat over a basin on the floor, but half an hour went by and nothing seemed to be happening. Then Neil started to fuss, and I put him to my breast. As soon as he began nursing, I felt a couple of sharp contractions and the placenta just plopped out into the basin."

Some physicians routinely remove the placenta manually right after the baby is born if the mother has an epidural in place for pain relief. There is no research to support this practice.

Researchers have studied the injection of saline solution or oxytocin into the umbilical cord vein to treat retained placenta, to try to avoid manual removal, but the results have been inconclusive.

Active Management of the Delivery of the Placenta

Some caregivers use "active management" of the third stage of labor. This combines the three components of giving oxytocin as soon as the baby is born, clamping the umbilical cord early and pulling on the cord to remove the placenta. Studies found that these three techniques, used together, produced a lower rate of postpartum hemorrhage and reduced the need for blood transfusions.

However, the studies are a bit confusing and it's not clear that all three steps are helpful. Giving oxytocin is the one element that is clearly associated with decreased risk of postpartum hemorrhage.

The Evidence About . . .
THE THIRD STAGE OF LABOR: DELIVERY OF THE PLACENTA

Giving oxytocin after the birth of the baby significantly reduces the risk of post-partum hemorrhage.

"Active management" of the third stage of labor still needs further research. It appears that routine oxytocin after delivery is more important than early cord clamping or traction on the cord in reducing the risk of postpartum hemorrhage.

If there is no unusual bleeding, waiting for up to an hour for the placenta to deliver will decrease the number of manual removals of the placenta that are performed without increasing the risk to the mother.

Part Five

Childbirth Challenges

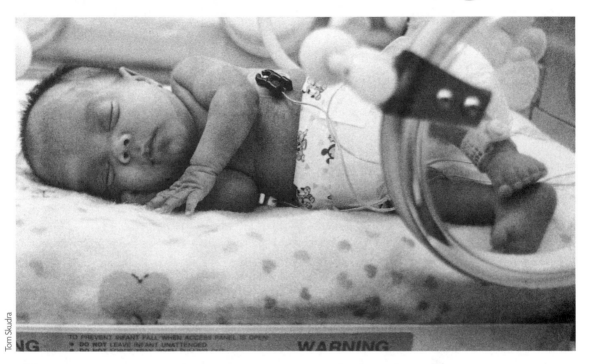

Tom Skudra

Most of the time, labor and birth are pretty straightforward. Sometimes, though, there are challenges. Perhaps you will go into labor when you are only seven months pregnant or, at the opposite end of the scale, find yourself two weeks past your due date and still waiting.

You may be thinking about having labor induced or wondering if you will need a Caesarean section to get this baby born. If you had a Caesarean with a previous baby, you might be wondering about giving birth vaginally this time. Knowing the results of the research studies can help you consider all your options in making these decisions.

Here's the best evidence about some of the more common challenges of childbirth, with information about Caesareans and why they are done, premature labor and birth, what it means to be "overdue" and more.

24

"Overdue?": Post-term Pregnancy

Lorna felt huge. Her "due date" had gone by two weeks ago, with no sign of a baby appearing. Two nights ago she'd had a dream about giving birth to a watermelon instead of a baby, and she was starting to wonder if labor would ever begin.

"I can't believe I'm actually eager to feel pain," she joked to a friend. "Every time I feel a twinge I keep hoping it will get worse and turn into good, hard contractions."

But when Lorna's doctor offered to induce her labor, Lorna surprised herself by saying no, she'd prefer to wait for labor to start on its own. Two days later, her water broke while she was sleeping, and her nine-pound baby girl was born seven hours later.

Lorna's pregnancy went longer than the average and is described by doctors as *prolonged*, *post-dates* or *post-term*. Until 30 years ago, prolonged pregnancy was not considered a problem that anything needed to be done about. People recognized that longer pregnancies led to bigger babies. Gradually, doctors also became aware that there was a slight increase in the rate of babies who died in labor or soon after birth if the pregnancy continued past 40 weeks. At that time, though, the risks to the baby were considered to be lower than the risks of intervening.

As an example of how recent the concerns about post-term pregnancy are, consider the changes in one medical textbook. *Williams Obstetrics*, a standard text, has had 19 editions since 1903. The 1997 edition is the *first* one to offer an entire chapter devoted to the post-term pregnancy.

Why is there so much interest in—and concern about—post-term pregnancy today?

First of all, researchers have now done a number of studies to analyze the risks of these longer-than-average pregnancies. Secondly, doctors now have safer methods of inducing labor, which make it less risky to intervene. Behind these two points, though, is the assumption that recognizing an increased risk means that intervention will be successful in preventing it.

The standard definition of a post-term pregnancy is 42 weeks, or 294 days from the first day of the woman's last menstrual period. This assumes that the baby was conceived two weeks after the day the period began. When the calculation is based on the mother's period, about 10 to 14 percent of pregnancies will be post-term.

This calculation isn't very reliable for women with irregular periods or longer-than-average menstrual cycles. When more accurate dating methods, such as ultrasound in early pregnancy or dating based on the woman's individual ovulation or conception time, are used, the number of post-term pregnancies is reduced to 3 to 4 percent.

There is a definite tendency for some mothers to have more than one post-term pregnancy, and for them to run in families, suggesting that sometimes prolonged pregnancies are genetic.

Julie said, "I went two weeks past my due date with Jason, and when the doctor suggested induction, I agreed. I spent a day on the drip and nothing happened, so I went home and told the doctor I'd changed my mind about being induced. Four days later, labor started and Jason was born. When I went past my due date again with Matthew, I decided to just wait. Sure enough, he was born at 42 ½ weeks. The funny thing is, my sister Tracey seems to have the same pattern."

What Are the Risks of Post-term Pregnancy?

Put bluntly, slightly more babies will die during labor or shortly after birth when the pregnancy continues past 42 weeks. Statistically, about 2.5 per 1000 infants born at 40 weeks (term) will die in labor or shortly after. At 42 weeks, about 4.5 per 1000 infants die. About 25 percent of these babies are abnormal, and

Things to Consider if You Are "Overdue"

- Are you certain of the dates of your last menstrual period?
- Are your menstrual cycles normally longer than 28 days, or are they irregular?
- Have you had an ultrasound to confirm the dates? When was it done? (It is only reliable for dating if done early in pregnancy.)
- Has the cervix begun to ripen? This has a big effect on how easy it will be to induce labor. (See Chapter 25, Induction of Labor.)
- Have any of your other pregnancies been longer than average but produced a healthy baby? This may suggest that longer pregnancies are typical for you.
- What are your "gut" feelings about being induced versus waiting?

would not have lived no matter when they were born. The rest usually die either from a lack of oxygen during labor or from meconium aspiration. Meconium is the dark, tarry substance in the baby's bowels before birth; if the baby has a bowel movement during or before labor, the meconium in the amniotic fluid can be inhaled into the baby's lungs and make the baby ill. This problem seems to be more common in babies born after 42 weeks.

Should You Be Induced?

For years, obstetricians have had different opinions on whether labor should be induced when a pregnancy becomes post-term. Early studies based on observation without control groups did not give any conclusive evidence.

In the meantime, routine induction of labor at or close to 42 weeks became very common.

More recently, some randomized studies have compared inducing labor at 40 weeks (term) with waiting for labor to start. Large randomized studies have looked at inducing labor at 41 weeks and compared this to waiting. No research has been done on pregnancies after 42 weeks. What did these studies find?

When the researchers compared inducing labor at 40 weeks to waiting for labor to begin spontaneously, they found no benefit or harm to mother or baby. Both groups had similar numbers of epidurals and Caesarean sections, and the babies had similar Apgar scores.

Induction of labor at 41 weeks versus waiting for labor was compared using a combined analysis of 11 separate studies. This is called a meta-analysis—and combining the results of studies in this way can give different results than if one big study is done. The researchers found little difference in the outcomes for the mothers. For the babies, there was no difference in fetal heart rate abnormalities or in depressed Apgar scores. However, there *was* a difference in perinatal death rates. One baby died in the group of women who had labor induced, versus nine deaths in a group of women who waited for the onset of labor.

This is a significant difference, and for this reason many doctors are recommending induction for all women at 41 weeks. However, a meta-analysis such as this should be viewed with caution, as the combined results of several small studies can be less reliable than one big study.

The authors of *Effective Care* suggest that induction should be *offered* to women at 41 weeks—in other words, each mother should make her own decision.

In all these studies, the "waiting for labor" group had some method of observation of the fetus used regularly—either non-stress testing, biophysical profile or fetal kick counting. These tests may predict pregnancies at higher risk, but there is minimal evidence that this information can be used to improve the outcome for the baby. If better ways to determine the well-being of the fetus are developed, and more effective methods of intervention are found, we may be able to further reduce the small risk of waiting for labor to start.

The Post-mature Baby

"Post-maturity" occurs in a small but unknown percentage of both full-term and post-term infants. Post-maturity is abnormal, and the name should not be used as a synonym for post-term pregnancy, which is usually just a variation of normal.

The post-mature infant has a unique and characteristic appearance. This includes wrinkled, patchy, peeling skin, particularly on the palms and soles, a long thin body and long fingernails. The baby typically is open-eyed and unusually alert, looking worried and "old." These babies are more likely to show signs of stress during labor, have decreased amounts of amniotic fluid and have meconium (the baby's first stool) in the amniotic fluid, and are more often stillborn.

Some of these post-mature infants are also post-term, but some are not. It may be that these infants have all experienced intra-uterine growth restriction at some stage of pregnancy. The majority of post-mature infants are not stillborn or asphyxiated at birth, and gain weight rapidly and do well after birth. There is no research to indicate that identifying these post-mature babies before birth and inducing labor reduces their risk of stillbirth and birth asphyxia.

The Evidence About...
"BEING OVERDUE"

Prolonged pregnancy is a variation of normal, and in the great majority of cases is associated with a good outcome for mother and baby. It may be part of a particular woman's biology and completely normal for her. However, prolonged pregnancy is also associated with a slightly increased risk to the baby.

Research combining 11 different studies (a meta-analysis) found that induction of labor at 41 weeks (compared to waiting for labor to begin on its own) lowered the perinatal death rate from 2.5 per 1000 to 0.3 per 1000.

Effective Care in Pregnancy and Childbirth suggests that at 41 weeks it is reasonable, in light of the present evidence, for the mother to make her own decision about whether she wants to be induced or to wait for labor to begin on its own.

25

Induction of Labor

Induction of labor is a deliberate attempt to start labor artificially, rather than waiting for it to start on its own. The most important thing about induction of labor is not how it will be done, but if it should be done at all. As obstetricians have found more effective methods to induce labor, the number of inductions has gone up considerably.

Induction of labor often seems very appealing. We are used to making appointments for important things, scheduling events into our daytimers and setting aside a certain block of time to do important tasks. We also tend to believe that it is good to "do something" rather than to be passive. The unpredictable nature of labor can be frustrating. Labor can start anytime three weeks before or after the "due date," and it can take from a couple of hours to a couple of days. This is not how we handle any other crucial happening in our lives, so planning the date of a baby's birth can seem like a good option. It's a reason mentioned by many women in choosing a repeat Caesarean over a VBAC, for example.

Induction can be helpful in some situations, but it is an intervention in the normal processes of pregnancy and birth, and like all interventions can bring its own problems.

The "outcomes" of inductions are not all measured in Caesarean section rates or number of babies needing resuscitation. A woman's confidence in her body's ability to labor and give birth normally is probably lessened if she is told that she "needs" to be induced. This suggests that her body is not working properly, and this lack of confidence may influence the progress of her labor.

Why Induce Labor?

The reasons given for inducing labor range from those that are lifesaving for mother or baby to those that are minor. You, your partner and your caregiver will need to decide which reasons make sense to you.

Sometimes the need for induction is clear. But when the reasons are not compelling, it is

Two "Optional" Inductions: Connie's Story

Connie never imagined she'd want to have labor induced, but in the end, she chose induction for both of her children.

"Both of my labors were induced. With my first pregnancy, I was a student. My boyfriend had left me halfway through the pregnancy. My mother, who has always been really close to me, had taken a month's leave of absence from her job so she could fly here and be with me when I had the baby. She came when I was 38 weeks, as my doctor had told me I could go into labor any time after that.

"At almost 42 weeks, we were still waiting! My mother had to fly home to go back to work in five days. We both went to my doctor's appointment that week. My mother is Dutch and she is really against interfering with pregnancy— she had me at home in Holland—but I couldn't imagine having the baby without her support. At my appointment, we asked about being induced.

"My doctor said that at 42 weeks induction was a very reasonable thing to consider, as it was certainly as safe for me and the baby as waiting. Then she suggested feeling my cervix to see if it was ripe—after she examined me, she said my cervix was really favorable and that she was sure the induction would work. By the time we left the office, both my mother and I were comfortable that an induction was what we wanted.

"The next day, I went into the hospital first thing in the morning. My doctor broke the water—I remember how warm it felt. The doctor said that the water was clear and that was a good thing. I walked around for half an hour dripping water and then the contractions started. I was really glad they started on their own because we had decided that if the contractions didn't start in four hours I would have an IV and Pitocin to start them, something I hoped to avoid. The rest of the labor and birth went fine.

"It was such a help to me to have my mother there—for me, that was more important than not being induced.

"With my next pregnancy, I was married. It turned out, though, that I was due right around the time my husband would have to be away on a course for work. When my due date got close, he kept putting off going to the course, but finally he was at the point where he had to go. This time I was only 40 weeks and five days. I remember exactly because I was counting!

"My husband really wanted to be here for the birth, and I really wanted him here as well. I talked it over with my doctor, and we agreed that even though this wasn't a medical reason, it was a reason that was important to us as a family.

"The induction went really well. I had hoped that just breaking the water would work again, but this time I only leaked a little bit of water and the contractions didn't start. My husband and I walked and walked all day, still no contractions. In the late afternoon, an IV and Pitocin were started. The contractions kicked in right away; within two hours, the doctor turned the Pitocin off and said my labor was on its own. Two hours later the baby was born.

"I'm really happy about both of my inductions, even though I am the type who would have told you that I would never be induced. Both times, the reasons were really important to me."

your preference (not your doctor's) that should be the deciding factor.

Reasons to induce labor are discussed below.

Illness in the Mother

The development or worsening of some disease in the mother completely unrelated to her pregnancy may be a reason for induction. Pregnant women can get cancer, thyroid disease, kidney disease and other medical conditions that need urgent treatment—but sometimes the treatment can't be started with the baby still in the uterus. Getting the baby born as soon as it can survive outside the uterus can allow the start of essential treatment for the mother.

Pre-eclampsia is an illness in the mother that is caused by pregnancy and threatens the safety of both mother and baby. With severe pre-eclampsia, the research is clear—the only cure is delivery of the baby. (Chapter 12, Hypertension and Pre-eclampsia, tells you more about this condition.)

Pre-labor Rupture of the Membranes

It is fairly common for the membranes containing the amniotic fluid to break before labor contractions start; usually this means that labor will start within the next few hours and that the baby will be born within the next day or two. Two to five percent of women who have this pre-labor rupture of the membranes, though, will still not have delivered their babies at the end of five days. The main concern when the membranes rupture long before the birth of the baby is an increased risk of infection in the mother and the newborn.

Research that compares waiting for labor after pre-labor rupture of the membranes with inducing labor *appears* to indicate that induction reduces the rate of infection in the newborn, but this may not be accurate. The diagnosis of infection in the newborn is difficult to make in the first hours after birth, so many babies are treated preventatively with antibiotics *simply because* the membranes were ruptured for a long time. When studies are done, these babies would then be classed as having been infected because they were on antibiotics. In reality, though, the babies may have been perfectly healthy.

Studies also found that induction of labor after spontaneous rupture of the membranes causes a longer and more painful labor and higher rates of Caesarean section. The risk of Caesarean section is less if prostaglandin is used for the induction, rather than oxytocin. The methods of inducing labor with these two drugs are described in more detail later.

Unusually Big or Small Babies

The baby who is bigger than average at term will sometimes be induced because of concerns that it will grow too big to deliver vaginally and will need a Caesarean section. Unfortunately, size alone does not predict which babies won't fit—the position of the baby's head in the pelvis is also important, as well as the strength of the labor. There is no evidence that inducing big babies at term is either beneficial or harmful.

Small babies raise different concerns. With the routine use of ultrasound, the diagnosis of the "small for dates" baby is made much more frequently. If the growth of the baby is seen to be less than average on a series of ultrasounds, induction may be recommended, on the basis that the environment inside the uterus is not nourishing the baby and it would grow better on the outside.

Unfortunately, the ultrasound can't always show the difference between babies who are suffering malnutrition in the uterus because of lack of circulation to the placenta, and therefore who would be better outside the uterus,

Robin's Induction: The Never-Ending Story

Robin's baby was "due" on February 22. That week at her appointment, her doctor examined her and said her cervix was thick and closed. On February 26, she had a biophysical profile, which showed the baby was doing well. On March 3, her doctor examined her again and told her that her cervix still wasn't ripe. She was now nine days overdue (41 weeks and two days) and her doctor told her he liked to induce everyone between 41 and 42 weeks. Robin says, "I didn't think anything of it. I just assumed that it was routine."

She was admitted to hospital that evening and had prostin gel put in her cervix. The next day an IV with Pitocin was started and ran all day. This only caused a few contractions, so the Pitocin was stopped at bedtime. Robin had another dose of prostin gel put in her cervix, and stayed in hospital for the second night. Another day on the Pitocin IV went by, and Robin still wasn't in labor.

That night the prostin gel treatment was repeated, but the next day the labor and delivery department was really busy. Robin says, "The nurse told me that they were too busy to run the Pitocin IV on me; then my doctor came in and told me I might as well go home and come back the next day to be induced again. I was really tired by then—I hadn't slept very well in the hospital. I hadn't had many real meals either, because they kept thinking I was going to be in labor so my meals didn't get ordered. Then they would realize I hadn't had anything to eat and get me a sandwich and juice."

Robin spent a night at home, then: "I went back the next day and the doctor said my cervix still wasn't ripe, so I had prostin gel put in every six hours all day long. I stayed overnight again, and the next day I had an Pitocin IV drip again and this time the doctor broke my water. I had what they called pit contractions all day, which sure hurt but didn't dilate my cervix very much. By supper-time I was so tired and in pain that I asked for an epidural—it worked great for the pain but I still couldn't really sleep because I was shaking and the nurses kept getting me to turn from side to side. Finally, early the next morning I had the baby. Of course, I was excited and happy, but I was so tired I couldn't think straight. It was days before I felt normal again, and I think a lot of it was lack of sleep."

Robin wishes she'd asked more questions and been more involved in the decision making. "When I look back, the decision to have the first dose of prostin gel was made so casually, and then things just kept going. It never occurred to me that I could have stopped it by just saying, 'this isn't working—let's stop and wait.' One thing just seemed to automatically lead to another, and I felt like I was on a merry-go-round I couldn't get off."

and babies who are just small and would benefit from more time in the uterus to grow.

Prolonged Pregnancy

Being "overdue" probably represents the major reason for induction of labor in North America. Prolonged pregnancy in most cases is a variation of normal and the baby does well regardless of whether the labor is induced or the mother waits for labor to start.

Very large comparisons of induction versus waiting have shown minimal differences in outcome for mothers or babies. Induction on the due date gives no advantage, while induction at 41 weeks appears to give a small increase in infant survival rates. (See Chapter 24, "Overdue?": Post-term Pregnancy.) Because outcomes are almost as good with waiting as with induction, the decision to induce should be made by the mother.

It's not always an easy decision. While some inductions are simple and straightforward, others become long, drawn-out, difficult procedures (see Robin's story in the previous sidebar, for example). Since inductions must be done in a hospital, women who have planned a home birth must come to terms with giving birth in hospital. Other women who had planned to have their babies in hospital but hoped to stay home as long as possible may be disappointed about going to the hospital before labor even starts and staying there through the whole process. Some women find this very stressful. Some studies have also found that women describe induced labors as more painful than labors that begin naturally.

Readiness of the Cervix: An Important Factor

The way the cervix feels at the beginning of the induction is the most important factor in predicting how the induction will proceed. If the cervix is unripe (meaning hard, long and closed), the induction is more likely to fail to start labor at all, labor is more likely to take a long time, and Caesarean section (because of a slow labor) is more likely. If the cervix is ripe (meaning soft, thin and starting to open), the induction is much more likely to go well.

Deciding whether the cervix is ripe or unripe is a subjective thing. A scoring system has been developed to describe the cervix, to try to make the evaluation more objective:

- *Consistency*: this describes whether the cervix feels hard or soft to the person doing the examination.

- *Effacement*: this measures the length of the cervix. During most of the pregnancy, the cervix is about 2 cm (0.8 in) long. Effacement describes how the cervix becomes shorter and flattens out to become an opening into the lower part of the uterus. Effacement is measured in percents—100 percent effaced means completely flattened out.

- *Position of the cervix*: this refers to whether the cervix is pointed down towards the mother's backbone or straight forward towards the opening of the vagina. The cervix pointing straightforward into the vagina is the most favorable.

- *Dilation*: this describes how open the cervix is; it is measured in centimeters or inches.

- *Position of the presenting part*: this refers to the position of the baby's head (or buttocks, if the baby is breech) in the mother's pelvis. The lower the baby's head, the likelier it is the induction will go well.

If the biggest part of the baby's head is lower than the mother's pubic bone, the baby is described as "engaged." For most white women having a first baby, the baby engages during the last few weeks of pregnancy, before labor starts; for later babies or for black women, the baby usually is not engaged until labor is underway. If your baby is engaged, induction is likely to be easier.

If the cervix is completely soft and 100 percent effaced, it is said to be ripe. If the cervix is also in the mid position in the vagina, if the baby's head is very low and if the cervix has started to dilate, these are the perfect conditions to do an induction.

If you are considering induction, it might help to know how ripe your cervix is. If it is very ripe, the induction will likely go well. If it is not ripe at all, you can predict that the induction may be more difficult, and you may want to rethink the idea.

Sometimes, induction is chosen even when the cervix is not ripe. As a result, methods to ripen it so that induction will be easier have been developed.

Artificial Ripening of the Cervix

Prostaglandins to Ripen the Cervix
Prostaglandins (prostins) are drugs that will ripen the cervix. A gel or tablet of prostin can be placed in the vagina, or the gel can be squeezed directly into the cervix. Prostaglandin ripening makes it more likely that the induction of labor will succeed. Labors with prostaglandin ripening also tend to be faster. In some cases, prostaglandin causes not just ripening of the cervix but the onset of labor as well.

If oxytocin is going to be used for the induction of labor, it should not be given until 6 to 12 hours after the prostaglandin ripening is done.

Very strong, frequent contractions and fetal heart rate abnormalities can occur during prostaglandin ripening. Despite this, the rate of Caesarean section and forceps or vacuum deliveries is lower in induced labors in which the cervix has been ripened with prostaglandin.

Mechanical Methods of Ripening the Cervix
The cervix may be ripened by inserting a balloon catheter into the cervix and blowing up the balloon. This is left in place, with the other end of the catheter taped to the mother's thigh, for 12 to 24 hours before the induction of labor. The steady pressure of the balloon on the cervix ripens the cervix, possibly by stimulating the release of natural prostaglandins. Other mechanical devices have also been used for the same purpose. The disadvantages of

these techniques are the pain of the insertion and a small risk of introducing infection. Research has found this method to be less effective in ripening the cervix than the prostaglandin gel.

Oxytocin to Ripen the Cervix
Oxytocin is a naturally occurring hormone that has been synthesized. While it is most often given to induce labor, it has also been given by intravenous drip over prolonged periods of time to ripen the cervix. Studies have shown that this method is unpleasant for the mother, can lead to water intoxication and is not very effective in actually ripening the cervix.

How Labor Is Induced

Methods used to induce labor include nipple stimulation, sweeping or rupturing the membranes or giving oxytocin or prostaglandin. Once again, induction of labor is more likely to succeed if the cervix is ripe.

Nipple Stimulation and Sexual Activity
Women have often been advised to stimulate their nipples, which causes oxytocin release, to start labor. Sex has also been recommended as a way of starting labor; during sexual intercourse prostaglandin is released from the cervix, and it is also present in semen. As can be imagined, the data to evaluate these methods come from rather small and uncontrolled studies! However, the research available suggests that nipple stimulation and regular sexual activity in late pregnancy do reduce the number of post-term pregnancies.

Women who are breastfeeding a baby or toddler while pregnant with the next baby are sometimes advised to wean, in case the older baby's suckling causes premature labor. There is no evidence that this can happen! Many women nurse through the pregnancy and continue, if they choose, to breastfeed both the older child and the new baby.

Lily became interested in these methods when she reached 41 weeks and her midwife discussed induction with her. "I didn't want to be induced if we could avoid it," Lily said, "and I figured sex and nipple stimulation couldn't hurt and would be fun even if it didn't work. I don't know if that's what did it, but after the third night of sex, I woke up at 3 a.m. in labor."

Sweeping the Membranes

Stripping or sweeping the membranes, also called a "stretch and sweep," has been a traditional method of inducing labor. The doctor or midwife inserts a finger through the cervix as far as possible and rotates it in a circle to separate the membranes from the wall of the lower part of the uterus. The limited data available suggest that stripping the membranes makes it more likely that the woman will go into labor within the next few days.

This technique is frequently used as an office procedure in post-term pregnancies to avoid formal induction. It is most easily and effectively performed if the cervix is ripe. Potential concerns are accidental rupture of the membranes and the introduction of infection.

Eleanor was five days past her due date when her doctor suggested trying a "stretch and sweep" at her regular prenatal appointment. "I was tired of being pregnant, and ready to try just about anything," Eleanor says. "It wasn't comfortable having it done, but it wasn't really painful. I went home feeling a bit funny—almost queasy—and by supper-time I was in labor. My doctor said it doesn't usually work that quickly, but I must have been ready to go."

Rupturing the Membranes

This is called artificial rupture of the membranes, breaking the water or amniotomy. It is done by putting an amni-hook (a long, thin, plastic stick with a small, sharp hook on its end) through the cervix and breaking the membranes with it. The membranes have no nerves, so it isn't painful—it just feels wet and warm as the fluid escapes.

Rupturing the membranes to induce labor has traditionally meant that you can't change your mind—once the membranes are ruptured, there is no turning back. The membranes are a barrier against infection in the uterus; once they are broken, it's easier for bacteria to get in. Since you have actually inserted something from outside (the amni-hook) into the membranes, the risk of infection is probably higher than if the membranes had ruptured on their own. However, caregivers differ on how long they feel a woman whose membranes have been ruptured artificially can safely wait until the baby is delivered, and this question has not been researched.

What if you rupture the membranes artificially and nothing happens—labor doesn't start? You can then be given oxytocin intravenously to induce labor. How long should you wait before receiving the oxytocin? There are no studies on this. Some doctors will start an oxytocin IV at the same time as they break the water; others will wait for a few hours, to see if anything happens.

A rare but very serious complication of rupture of the membranes is the umbilical cord slipping through the cervix (cord prolapse). The cord is then between the baby's head and the cervix, and will be compressed when the uterus contracts, cutting off the circulation to the baby. This is an emergency requiring immediate Caesarean section. A cord prolapse is more likely to occur if the membranes are ruptured before the baby's head is well down into the mother's pelvis.

Oxytocin IV

Oxytocin is the most widely used method to induce labor. Oxytocin (sometimes called Pitocin or "the pit drip") is given by IV at a carefully regulated rate, which is gradually increased until regular contractions result. Once labor begins, the rate of oxytocin infusion usually doesn't need to be increased; frequently, the rate of the infusion can actually be reduced or even be stopped altogether as active labor "kicks in."

Oxytocin can sometimes induce very strong contractions, causing the baby to be stressed, and, rarely, causing rupture of the uterus. There has been a tendency to use continuous electronic fetal monitoring for all labors induced with oxytocin. Research to support this practice has not been done. In any case, continuous monitoring does not replace careful attention by a bedside nurse. The frequency and strength of contractions can change very quickly with a small change in the dose of oxytocin.

Studies suggest that oxytocin induction without rupture of the membranes will not start labor in about one-third of cases. Oxytocin plus artificial rupture of membranes is more likely to establish labor within a few hours than oxytocin alone. With this combination approach, though, the doctor generally commits to having the baby born within a definite time limit, often 24 hours. Labor not progressing this quickly will lead to delivery by Caesarean section. If the membranes have **not** been ruptured and the oxytocin induction doesn't work, the mother can choose to go home and try another day.

Prostaglandins

The ability of prostaglandins to ripen the cervix has already been discussed. In some women, prostaglandin used to ripen the cervix also made them go into labor. Prostaglandin gel in the vagina has been investigated as a method of inducing labor. Repeat doses of prostaglandin can be used, usually every 6 to 12 hours.

Kendra says, "When my doctor told me she wanted to induce me and that she planned to use the oxytocin drip, I asked her about the prostaglandin gel. She said she didn't normally use it, but when I told her what I'd read—that it tends to make induction more successful—she said we could certainly give it a try.

"The plan was to put in the gel in the morning, then start the oxytocin later that day. My doctor inserted the gel, then left for the office, saying she'd come back around noon. Well, my contractions started almost immediately and I had a fast, intense labor. The nurses had to call the doctor back—my baby was born at 11:30! We were very pleased that we decided to use the gel."

Prostaglandin is easier to use than oxytocin because no intravenous is required, so women can walk around freely. Prostaglandin can be used whether the membranes are ruptured or not.

How does prostaglandin compare with oxytocin for inducing labor? Doctors have much more experience with oxytocin, which has been used widely for 40 years, than with prostaglandin, which is a newer drug. Studies comparing the two drugs have only included small numbers of women so far. In the studies that exist, though, the number of women who deliver within 12 hours of induction is the same with both methods. However, after 24 and 48 hours, there are more women who have given birth in the prostaglandin group than in the oxytocin group. Caesarean section rates are very slightly lower in the prostaglandin group, and rates of forceps and vacuum deliveries are significantly lower in the prostaglandin group. There were no significant differences seen in outcomes for the babies.

Are Induced Labors More Painful?

There is a widely held belief that induced labor is more painful than spontaneous labor. Certainly, women who describe their induced labors often comment on the pain, and women who have had both induced and naturally starting labors will often say that the induction was more painful.

Despite this, the incidence of epidural anesthesia is the same in the two groups. This is surprising, given that induced women are in hospital during their whole labor, and that inductions are carried out during daylight hours: two factors that make anesthesia very available to the induced women, and might have made it more likely that they would use it.

A different use of oxytocin is to make a slowly progressing labor faster by making the contractions stronger and closer together—this is called augmenting the labor. Not surprisingly, women also perceive this as more painful than the labor to that point, and epidural use is more common with augmented labors.

Caesarean Section Rates and Induced Labor

Many people also believe that induction causes a higher Caesarean section rate than spontaneous labor. This is undoubtedly true. How-ever, many inductions are done because of problems with the mother or baby that make delivery necessary. In these cases, the induction is an alternative to Caesarean section, not an alternative to waiting for spontaneous labor. If the induction isn't effective, or doesn't move things along quickly enough, a Caesarean becomes necessary. It is impossible to separate the risk of Caesarean section caused by induction itself from the risk caused by the *reason* for the induction being done in the first place.

Talking to Your Doctor about Inducing Labor

If your doctor suggests that you have your labor induced, it's very important that you know the reasons for the induction. If induction is suggested because you are "overdue," for example, you might want to go over the information in Chapter 24, "Overdue?": Post-term Pregnancy. If you have pregnancy-induced hypertension, read Chapter 12, Hypertension and Pre-eclampsia. This will help you to make a more informed decision.

Ask your doctor what could happen if you decide not to be induced. If there isn't an emergency situation, consider trying some of the natural methods of encouraging labor to start first.

The Evidence About . . .
INDUCTION OF LABOR

Induction of labor is a good treatment for complications in which the baby will be better off born than remaining in the uterus.

Ripening of the cervix increases the chance that the induction will succeed, that labor will be shorter and that the baby will be born vaginally. The best method of ripening the cervix is prostaglandin gel applied to the cervix.

Combining oxytocin and rupturing the membranes is more likely to be successful in inducing labor than either alone.

Prostaglandins used to induce labor appear more likely than oxytocin to result in vaginal birth within a reasonable length of time after starting the induction, and to lower the rate of vacuum, forceps or Caesarean delivery. This information, though, is based on very small studies.

Although induction is easy to attempt, this does not mean it should be done. If induction is recommended, think about the reasons for doing it first, before considering how it will be done.

26

When the Water Breaks before Labor Starts: Pre-labor Rupture of the Membranes

During pregnancy, the developing baby floats inside a bag of fluid known as the amniotic sac. The membranes holding the amniotic fluid usually break sometime during labor (although some babies are born with the membranes still intact, and in many cultures this is considered a sign of good luck). Sometimes the membranes break before labor starts. This is called *pre-labor rupture of the membranes*, or PROM.

If your membranes rupture, you might feel or hear a "pop," or you might not feel anything except the gush or trickle of warm water from your vagina. At first, women often don't realize they are leaking amniotic fluid; they think they've lost control of their bladders. Sometimes the fluid drips out in small, hardly noticeable amounts; other women have water running down their legs in substantial quantities. There may be an initial gush followed by a slower, steady trickle, or there may be periodic gushes of water once contractions begin.

Alana woke up one morning (a week after her due date) thinking she had heard a noise in the bedroom. When she sat up in bed, she real-ized what that noise had been: her membranes had ruptured and the mattress was now soaked.

Louanne arrived at the hospital when her contractions were five minutes apart. The nurse who examined her asked, "When did your water break? I can't feel any membranes here." Thinking it over, Louanne said it might have happened just before labor started, when she thought she had leaked a little urine. "It was hardly anything," she says, "so I didn't realize that it might have been my water breaking."

In 70 percent of women, labor will start soon after the membranes rupture and their babies will be born within 24 hours. Ninety percent of women will give birth within 48 hours of their membranes rupturing. Another 5 to 8 percent will have their babies within the next couple of days, but 2 to 5 percent will still be waiting to give birth five days after the membranes rupture.

Why is this wait a concern? Because without the membranes present to act as a barrier, it's easier for germs to get into the uterus and cause an infection that could make the mother and/or the baby ill.

Pre-labor Rupture of the Membranes Pre-term

Christina was just six months pregnant when she noticed a steady trickle of fluid from her vagina. She called her midwife, who suggested she go immediately to the hospital because her baby was so premature. Contractions had started in earnest by the time she arrived, and progressed quickly once in hospital. Emily was born weighing a little less than three pounds. "It took me by surprise," Christina says. "It was pretty frightening to go through, not knowing how the baby would be."

After a lengthy stay in the neonatal intensive care unit, baby Emily came home weighing five pounds and is a healthy, active little girl.

Rupture of the membranes when the baby is premature (before 37 weeks) and before labor has started is called pre-term pre-labor rupture of the membranes.

When pre-labor rupture of the membranes occurs pre-term, the mother will likely go into labor, usually right away, and almost always within a week. Research shows that it does not improve the outcome for the baby to use drugs to try to delay the labor, to try to stop labor once it starts or to induce labor (unless there are signs of infection). Giving the mother antibiotics during the time she is waiting for labor to start can reduce the risk of infection in mother and baby. (See Chapter 28, Premature Labor and Birth.)

Pre-labor Rupture of the Membranes at Term

Christina had extra concerns because her baby was premature. In most cases, though, the membranes rupture when the baby is full-term and ready to be born. Labor contractions usually start within a few hours.

Vicky was walking home from the park in the early afternoon with her toddler in the stroller, when she felt a familiar gush of water between her legs. This had happened to her twice before—right at 40 weeks, her water broke before her contractions started. The previous two times, her doctor had urged her to go to the hospital immediately, even though she wasn't having any contractions. Once at the hospital, she was given oxytocin to induce labor, hooked up to a fetal monitor and went through many hours of hard contractions before giving birth.

During this pregnancy, just in case it happened again, Vicky had done some research. She had seen studies that suggested the rates of Caesarean section and anesthetic in labor were higher when women with pre-labor rupture of the membranes were induced. The research found that the rate of infection was no higher if women simply waited to go into labor normally. Some of the research suggested that the risk of infection could be reduced if the woman stayed at home rather than going to the hospital to be examined internally. (Her body would already be resistant to most of the familiar germs at home, while the wider variety of germs at the hospital would be more dangerous.)

Vicky decided not to call her doctor this time and simply stayed home, leaking a little fluid throughout the evening. She had a shower rather than a bath, and she changed the sanitary pads she was wearing as soon as they became wet. Shortly after midnight, she began having contractions. At that point, she woke up her husband and they headed to the hospital. Her baby was born four hours later.

"It was my best, easiest labor," Vicki says. "I would do the same thing if it happened again.

I'm not sure exactly how long I would wait, but I definitely would not agree to be induced as soon as my water broke."

Studies found that the total length of time from the moment the membranes ruptured to the moment the baby was born was shorter when labor was induced (an average of 24 hours, compared to 30 hours when labor was allowed to start on its own). But the length of *actual labor* averaged 15 hours with induction, compared to only six hours for the women who waited for labor to begin spontaneously.

The mother who is induced with oxytocin immediately after her water breaks may experience a harder and longer labor and an increased risk of Caesarean section to deliver her baby than if she just waits. If an induction is done, the risk of Caesarean section is lower when prostaglandin is used to induce rather than oxytocin.

Will Inducing Labor Reduce the Baby's Chance of Getting an Infection?

Concerns about infection have been the main reason for encouraging induction of labor once the membranes have ruptured. However, there is no good research to support this approach. Other factors need to be included in future studies: staying at home versus going to the hospital (where there are more germs), number of vaginal exams, etc. More research is needed in this area.

Studies done in the 1960s compared giving all mothers with pre-labor rupture of the membranes antibiotics versus only giving antibiotics if there were early signs of infection (these

---

The Evidence About...
PRE-LABOR RUPTURE OF THE MEMBRANES

Rupture of the membranes before the start of labor at term is a normal event; no good data are available for how often it happens.

Once membranes rupture, 90 percent of women will deliver spontaneously within 48 hours.

Women with prolonged rupture of the membranes before delivery at term may have a higher risk of infection for themselves and their babies, but it is uncertain whether this risk of infection can be reduced by inducing labor rather than waiting for labor to start on its own.

Pre-term pre-labor rupture of the membranes almost always leads to premature birth. Administration of antibiotics while waiting for labor and during labor reduces maternal and fetal infections. There is no benefit to trying to stop premature labor once the membranes have ruptured.

---

signs include a slight fever in the mother and a rapid heartbeat in the baby). There were no benefits to routine antibiotics for the babies. On the other hand, the mothers who received routine antibiotics did develop fewer infections after this preventive treatment.

27

Problems with the Amniotic Fluid

Your baby floats in your uterus in a pool of amniotic fluid contained in a sac or membrane. Amniotic fluid is normally clear or very pale yellow. The average amount of amniotic fluid by term is about 1 liter (1.06 quarts), but volume ranges tremendously in normal pregnancies with healthy babies. A very large amount or a very small amount of amniotic fluid can be associated with bad outcomes, but there is a large overlap between normal and abnormal volumes. You will have the most amniotic fluid at about 36 weeks; the amount then gradually decreases over the final few weeks.

Too little amniotic fluid is called *oligohydramnios*. This is a difficult diagnosis to make, as small volumes of fluid are hard to measure, even with ultrasound. From 15 to 25 percent of cases of low fluid volume are caused by abnormal fetuses. If you have very little amniotic fluid, your baby is more likely to show signs of distress in labor. Fetal heart rate abnormalities during labor frequently occur with oligohydramnios, because the lack of cushioning from the fluid makes it easier for

the umbilical cord to be compressed, cutting down the oxygen supply to the baby.

When there is an unusually large amount of amniotic fluid, it is called *polyhydramnios*—defined as 2 liters (2.12 quarts) or more of amniotic fluid. About 1 woman out of 100 has polyhydramnios, and most of the time there is no known cause. Polyhydramnios is associated with a higher-than-average rate of premature labor, premature separation of the placenta and postpartum hemorrhage. As well as these serious complications, it can be extremely uncomfortable for the mother.

"People kept asking me if I was having twins," Caroline remembers. "I knew I wasn't, but it was obvious that I was much larger than the other women in my prenatal class. When labor started and my water broke, the reason became obvious—it was like Niagara Falls!"

Meconium in the Amniotic Fluid

Meconium is the baby's first bowel movement.

About 80 percent of babies do not pass meconium until after they are born. That leaves 20 percent who will have this first bowel movement while they are still inside the uterus, either before or during labor. When there is meconium in the amniotic fluid, the baby is at a greater risk of potentially serious complications. The baby may inhale some of the meconium before labor, during labor or as it is being born, and this can cause pneumonia.

If your membranes rupture in labor (or are deliberately broken by your caregiver), you may notice that the fluid looks yellowish, medium green or dark green, depending on how much stool the baby has passed and how long ago it was passed.

If there is a lot of meconium and little amniotic fluid at the beginning of labor, the risk to the baby is significant. On the other hand, if you have a normal amount of amniotic fluid but you see a slight yellow staining, there is probably little risk to your baby. It is unusual for a baby to pass meconium for the first time in labor (unless the baby is breech), and this may mean it is in distress.

Considering how often meconium is seen in the amniotic fluid (20 percent of the time), there have been very few studies to test different methods of managing these labors.

Unless the membranes have ruptured, you won't even know if you have meconium in the amniotic fluid. Some physicians have suggested that every laboring woman should have her membranes ruptured as soon as she arrives at the hospital, so that the doctor can check for meconium. Alternately, the doctor or nurse could use an amnioscope to look through the vagina and cervix to assess the amniotic fluid without breaking the membranes. Neither of these suggestions has ever been researched, so it is impossible to say whether they would improve outcomes for the baby.

Amnioinfusion

Some small research studies have tested *amnioinfusion* on mothers in labor. Amnioinfusion is a technique of adding intravenous fluids to the uterus to increase the volume of amniotic fluid and dilute the meconium. In several studies, this treatment seemed to reduce the number of babies who developed problems from inhaling meconium.

Amnioinfusion has also been studied in cases where the mother has very small amounts of amniotic fluid. Babies in this situation often have heart rate abnormalities during labor. Amnioinfusion decreased the heart rate abnormalities; more importantly, it also decreased Caesarean section rates, the number of babies asphyxiated at birth, low Apgar scores and low umbilical artery pH at birth.

It must be noted that these trials have been performed on small numbers of women, and that they have been carried out at major teaching institutions by researchers skilled in the techniques. However, if you are having your baby at a large teaching hospital, and are concerned because you have little amniotic fluid, it would be worth asking your doctor if this treatment is available to you.

Treating the Baby

When there is meconium in the amniotic fluid, the risk of the baby breathing it in at birth and getting pneumonia possibly can be reduced by suctioning the baby's mouth and nose immediately after birth. This is done virtually routinely, even though its usefulness in preventing aspiration pneumonia is unproven. Too vigorous suctioning deep in the baby's throat can cause slow heart rate and impair the baby's breathing.

Suctioning of the trachea (windpipe) for infants who have passed meconium before birth is a much more difficult and dangerous procedure, requiring that a small tube be inserted into the trachea. Risks include injury to the throat or windpipe, slow heart rate, reduced oxygen supply to the baby, collapse of the lung and infection. This procedure has not been tested in randomized studies.

This procedure may be beneficial if it is used *only* for babies who are born with very thick meconium present and who are showing signs of distress.

The Evidence About...
AMNIOTIC FLUID

When the amount of amniotic fluid is too high or too low, the baby is more likely to have problems. In most cases, though, these problems are not treatable. Amnioinfusion may help when there is too little fluid.

If the baby has a bowel movement before birth, it may be a sign of stress. The baby may also inhale some of the meconium (the pre-birth bowel movement) and become seriously ill as a result. Suctioning the baby's mouth and nose as it is born is the usual treatment for this; although it has not been studied, it seems to be safe.

28

Premature Labor and Birth

Brenda was at home alone when she noticed that the cramps she'd been feeling all day were getting stronger and more regular. Finally she called her sister-in-law, who already had two children, and described the odd pains she was feeling.

"I hate to say this, Brenda," her sister-in-law said, "but I think you're in labor."

"I can't be in labor," said Brenda. "I'm not even seven months pregnant!"

But Brenda was, in fact, in labor and she gave birth to a three-pound baby girl later that night. Her daughter spent nearly eight weeks in the special-care nursery of the hospital. At age six, complications from her prematurity continue to affect her walking and her speech.

Not all babies born prematurely will be disabled as Brenda's daughter is, of course, but many are. Premature birth is a major cause of death among babies, and a major cause of disability among children who survive being born too early.

Premature or Just Small?

The premature baby is born before 37 complete weeks of pregnancy. The length of time inside the uterus is more important here than the baby's weight, as some premature babies are considerably larger than others.

Shannon, for example, gave birth to her son when she was 34 weeks pregnant. He weighed 5 lbs. 9 oz. Even though he had arrived early, he was large for his gestational age. Despite his bigger-than-average size, he did have some of the other problems common in premature babies: he developed respiratory distress syndrome (breathing problems) and occasional spells of apnea (when he would stop breathing altogether). However, he soon overcame these problems and was able to go home with his family after three weeks in a special-care nursery.

Babies who are born between 34 and 37 weeks are premature, but they are almost as likely to survive and be healthy as full-term babies. They usually only need some extra help in staying warm, in getting enough calories to grow and in learning to nurse in the first few weeks. There isn't much point, then, in trying to stop labor if the mother is more than 34 weeks pregnant. Research on premature labor and birth, therefore, has concentrated on situations where the mother is less than 34 weeks pregnant.

Lots of research has been done on premature babies born between 26 and 34 weeks, and the survival rates for this group have increased tremendously. Newborn intensive care has also made possible the survival of some infants of less than 26 weeks gestation and with very low birth weights (below 1000 grams—about 2 pounds).

"When I first saw John, I couldn't imagine that he would survive," says Marjorie. "I remember that he was so small that my husband Jack could cradle his whole body in the palm of his hand. But the nurses said he was a fighter, and he made it."

But while Jack and Marjorie were thrilled that John survived his very premature birth, they also had to contend with the complications. John needed surgery before he was a month old, and had two more operations before his first birthday. He is deaf and developmentally delayed. Disabilities and various health problems are more common in these very small babies.

Can We Prevent Premature Labor before It Starts?

There has been great interest in trying to predict early in pregnancy the 10 percent of women who will go into premature labor, with the hope that a treatment can be discovered to prevent it.

The risk factors listed in the sidebar are sometimes used as a scoring system to pre-

Some Factors that Make Premature Birth More Likely

- Mother has already had a premature baby.
- Mother is less than 20 years old.
- Family is poor and food is inadequate.
- Mother smokes.
- Mother drinks or uses recreational drugs heavily.
- Mother has a chronic disease such as hypertension or diabetes.
- Mother is carrying twins, triplets or other multiples.
- The baby has serious birth defects.
- Mother's blood pressure has become high during the pregnancy.
- The placenta has separated from the uterus, or is covering the cervix.
- The baby has intra-uterine growth restriction.
- There is an infection in the uterus.

dict which women will deliver prematurely, but it hasn't turned out to be very reliable. At least half of the women who give birth prematurely will not have any of the risk factors on the list.

However, women with high scores on this list *are* more likely to have premature births, and this has given researchers a group to work with. Several treatments to prevent premature labor and birth before it starts have been studied.

Social Interventions
When women live in poverty and don't get enough food, they have a higher chance of giving birth prematurely. Several programs have tried to improve the situations of these pregnant women by providing additional food or improved living conditions, but none has

reduced the number of premature births. It may be that this support must start long before pregnancy to be helpful.

Bed Rest

Bed rest has *not* been demonstrated to be effective in preventing premature birth.

Suturing the Cervix Closed

Suturing the cervix closed (called cervical cerclage) in early pregnancy and releasing it at term has been used to attempt to prevent premature birth. The mother needs an anesthetic for this procedure. For most women considered to be at risk of premature birth, the procedure did not make any difference. The only benefit from cervical cerclage was seen in a very small group of women who had already had three premature births.

Checking the Cervix During Pregnancy

With this approach, women who were felt to be at risk of premature birth were seen frequently during their pregnancies. At each visit a pelvic examination was performed and the cervix was felt to see if it was softening and effacing (getting shorter), or starting to dilate. Ultrasound was used to measure the length of the cervix in some of these women. Women with significant effacement and dilation of the cervix during their pregnancy *are* at higher risk for premature labor, but this knowledge did not lead to any improvement in the rate of premature birth.

Home Monitoring of Uterine Activity

Research studies have given some women small recorders that attached by straps around their abdomens. They wear these as they go about their normal daily routines, and the device keeps track of any contractions of the uterus. Once a day, the woman calls a phone number the doctor has given her and attaches the recorder to the phone to download the information. This method is very expensive, and, at this point, does not seem to reduce the number of premature births.

Medications

Women considered to be at high risk have been given several different drugs during their pregnancy to prevent premature labor, including ritodrine, magnesium, calcium, progesterone and antibiotics. None of them have reduced the number of premature births.

To summarize, these methods have all been tried with women who were not in labor, but who were felt to be at high risk of premature labor. None of these methods has been particularly effective in preventing premature birth.

Can We Stop Premature Labor once It Starts?

It sounds simple: stop premature labor and you'll prevent premature births. But the situation isn't quite that black and white.

Not all premature labor leads to premature birth. You might be 30 weeks pregnant and experience painful contractions for six hours; then they stop and your pregnancy continues until you are full-term. Yes, you experienced premature labor, but it was a false labor that was going to stop anyway. If you had gone to the hospital and been treated with medication, you might have given the drug the credit for stopping your labor and preventing the premature birth of your baby.

Also, stopping premature labor does not necessarily prevent premature birth. You might go into labor at 28 weeks, have it stopped with drugs and then give birth to a premature baby a week later. The treatment worked at the time, but you still had a premature baby.

For these reasons, randomized controlled

studies are exceedingly important in assessing interventions to stop premature *labor*, to see if they actually prevent premature *birth*. To assess any treatment proposed for the prevention of premature labor, it is essential to have a control group of women with the same symptoms and signs of labor who are untreated.

The first challenge researchers face is deciding whether a woman is actually in labor. The earlier in labor that an intervention is started, the better the chances are of stopping labor. But it is in the earliest stages that it is hardest to know whether you are actually in labor or not; contractions come and go, with some being strong and some being weak. Most researchers have arbitrarily defined pre-term labor as regular contractions (at least every five to eight minutes) that have produced 80 percent effacement or 2 cm (0.8 in) dilation of the cervix.

Many different methods of stopping premature labor have been tested in clinical trials. None of them have proven effective at actually preventing premature births.

The most useful drugs appear to be the betamimetic drugs (Ritodrine and Terbutaline). These drugs relax the uterus and have been shown to reduce the numbers of babies born 24 and 48 hours after starting treatment. But the drugs don't reduce the number of infant deaths or the number of babies with respiratory distress syndrome. There are several possible reasons for this. The drugs do have some complications, which may balance out the benefits. And they appear to stop labor only temporarily, so that the baby may still be born prematurely. This temporary delay, though, can be very valuable when the time gained is used to arrange the best possible conditions for the baby's birth. Read on.

Helping the Baby's Lungs to Mature

The most serious risk to premature babies is respiratory distress syndrome (RDS). Fifty percent of the babies born before 34 weeks will have this problem. Babies with RDS breathe very hard and fast, and despite their struggles, often can't get enough oxygen. They are either given extra oxygen to breathe or, in serious cases, attached to a machine called a ventilator that breathes for them.

Corticosteroid drugs, given to the mother in premature labor, can cut her baby's risk of RDS in half. The maximum benefit to the baby's lungs is achieved if the baby is born within one to seven days after the treatment is completed, but there are still benefits if the baby is born sooner or later than that.

The use of betamimetic drugs to delay the birth allow time for corticosteroids to be given to the mother.

Corticosteroid treatment in premature labor also reduces the risk of two other complications of the first week of life for premature babies: bleeding into the brain and serious inflammation of the bowel.

In pregnancies where the only complication is prematurity, corticosteroid drugs don't cause any side effects. In premature labors where there are other complications as well, the situation is less clear-cut. Particularly in pregnancies with high blood pressure, intra-uterine growth restriction and diabetes, the risks and benefits of corticosteroids appear about equal.

When Should Premature Labor Be Allowed to Continue?

Stopping premature labor is not always the best thing. In some cases, doctors have suggested that premature labor is nature's way of removing the baby from a uterus that is not nourishing it properly. There are some situations where it may be best for the mother and/or the baby that premature birth occur.

For example, if there is a severe infection of the uterus, mother and baby will be better off if the baby is born quickly and they are both treated with antibiotics. When the mother has hypertension and/or a growth-restricted infant, premature labor may be welcomed, as there is concern about the safety of the baby inside the uterus.

In fact, in pregnancies complicated by conditions such as hypertension, diabetes or Rh problems, premature labor may be deliberately planned and induced. Planned, elective pre-term deliveries represent about one-quarter of all premature births. In these situations, it is felt that the risk of being born prematurely is less than the risk of more time in the uterus exposed to the complicating disease.

Pre-labor Rupture of the Membranes (PROM) Pre-term

If your water breaks before labor starts, the medical term for this is pre-labor rupture of the membranes, or PROM. When this happens before you are 37 weeks pregnant, it is PROM pre-term. Most women give birth within a week of the membranes rupturing, so your risk of having a premature baby at this point is high.

There is also a risk that bacteria will get into the uterus from the vagina and the baby will become infected. This risk is greater the more premature the baby is. As well, there is increased risk of prolapse of the umbilical cord, either at the time of the rupture or at the start of labor. Separation of the placenta from the wall of the uterus is also more common,

because of the sudden decrease in the size of the uterus as the amniotic fluid flows out.

Several different methods of treatment of the woman with PROM pre-term have been studied.

Preventive Antibiotics
Antibiotics given to the mother, either before labor starts or during labor, will reduce the infection rate for both mother and baby. However, antibiotics don't change the number of babies who do not survive. This is hard to explain, unless the studies simply have not been big enough to show an effect on a rare event like death.

Corticosteroids
Giving corticosteroids to improve lung maturity has the same benefit with ruptured membranes as without, a 50 percent decrease in the incidence of respiratory distress syndrome in the newborn. There is no increased risk of infection.

Induction of Labor
Studies comparing induction of labor with waiting to see what happens after PROM pre-term showed no benefit from induction of labor.

Waiting
Waiting to see what happens, while carefully observing the mother and baby, seems to be a safe approach with PROM pre-term. If labor starts, as it usually does, there is no benefit to trying to stop it. Sometimes labor does not start, the membranes seal themselves again, the fluid reaccumulates and the pregnancy continues to term.

That's what happened to Elaine. "At seven months, I thought I'd lost control of my bladder. When I went to the doctor, she told me that my membranes had ruptured and I'd better get to the hospital because I was probably going to have a premature baby.

"I was surprisingly calm as we headed to the hospital. I think it was because I wasn't having any contractions, so the possibility of giving birth soon didn't seem real to me. After discussing different options with my doctor and my husband, we decided to just wait.

"Within 48 hours, the dripping had stopped. My doctor told me that the membranes seemed to have resealed, and sent me home the next day. I ended up going past my due date and we were starting to talk about induction before I went into labor! I thought that was pretty funny when two months earlier we'd been worried about a premature baby."

Place of Birth

The safest place for a very premature infant to be delivered is in a specialized center with a newborn intensive care nursery. This center will have expertise in caring for any complications in the mother, as well as neonatalogists (pediatricians who specialize in premature infants) available around the clock to attend the birth and subsequently care for the baby in the nursery.

If you go into labor prematurely, decisions will need to be made. Your community hospital may have the equipment and expertise to take care of your baby if you are 35 weeks pregnant, but if you are only 31 weeks pregnant (or less), your doctor might advise transferring you to a specialized center for your birth. How far along you are in your labor and how far away the other hospital is will determine if transfer before the birth is possible. If labor is too advanced and there is no time for transfer to the specialized center, the baby may be born and initially treated in the community hospital and then transferred (if

The Neonatal Intensive Care Unit (NICU)

If your baby is premature (or sick) she will probably be cared for in an NICU. For parents, this can be an intimidating place.

- A nurse will be assigned to care for your baby (and probably one or two other babies as well).
- Lab technicians and X-ray technicians will perform tests on your baby.
- One doctor will be the primary caregiver for your baby, but she will also be examined and treated by others.
- A ward clerk will handle paperwork and phone calls.
- The incubator is a heated glass box that allows your baby to be easily observed. She will probably be wearing just a diaper, or a diaper and a hat.
- Oxygen can be piped into the incubator or given to the baby through a mask or nasal tube.
- If your baby needs help in breathing, a respirator may be used. A tube goes through your baby's nose and into her lungs, and connects to a machine beside her incubator.
- Your baby may have an intravenous line inserted in a vein in her hand, foot or scalp.
- An electrode to keep track of your baby's heart rate and oxygen level is attached as well–often wrapped around her foot.
- A thermometer to measure your baby's temperature may be taped to her abdomen.
- Many of these machines make beeping noises or have flashing lights, and if several go off at once it can be scary.

necessary) to the specialized center for continuing care.

The betamimetic drugs that temporarily stop labor can buy some time here—time to be transferred to a hospital with a special-care nursery, and time to be given the corticosteroids that will help your baby's lungs mature.

Preventing the Complications of Premature Birth

When prevention hasn't worked, and it is obvious that the labor is going to continue and you are going to deliver a premature baby, there are some special things to think about.

An ultrasound examination can be helpful. Ultrasound shows your doctor the position of the baby. Because premature babies haven't had time to settle into the normal head-down position of the full-term baby, your baby is more likely to be lying crosswise or in a breech (bottom-first) position. An ultrasound also will check to see if the placenta is overlapping the cervix. With the ultrasound information to help, your doctor can discuss the best approach to your baby's birth with you.

You will probably be offered corticosteroids to help prevent respiratory distress syndrome. Your baby's risk of infection can also be decreased if you are given antibiotics while you are in labor.

Many premature babies have bleeding into their brain. The more premature the baby is, the more common and serious this is. Some studies have found that giving the drug phenobarb or vitamin K to the mother during labor has reduced this risk, but more research on this is needed.

Slowing of the fetal heart rate is frequently seen during premature labor, especially when the membranes have ruptured before labor begins. This is possibly due to the umbilical cord being compressed once there is less amniotic fluid to provide a cushioning effect. If a small tube is inserted through the cervix into the uterus, fluid can be infused into the uterus. This is called amnioinfusion. No definite conclusions about whether this is helpful in premature labors can be made based on the current evidence.

Will a Caesarean Section Prevent Complications?

Should your premature baby be delivered vaginally or by Caesarean section? We don't have good evidence to say that delivery by Caesarean is safer for all premature babies or for specific groups of premature babies (such as those in a breech position, or those who are very small). Since Caesarean sections have significant risks for the mother, the decision should not be made lightly.

While some studies have found a higher survival rate for premature babies by Caesarean section when compared to those delivered vaginally, the two groups compared were not the same. Some of the mothers who delivered vaginally had babies who were considered too small or too ill to be delivered by Caesarean section. Others were too far along in labor to arrange for a Caesarean. These mothers in advanced labor also didn't have time to be given corticosteroid drugs, or to arrange for a neonatologist to be present at the delivery.

Can Interventions in Vaginal Births Prevent Complications?

A number of interventions have commonly been recommended when premature babies are born vaginally, and are routine in many places. Considering how many babies are born prematurely, it is surprising that these interventions have not been more extensively studied. However, the small studies that have

Kangaroo Care

Research by Dr. Anthony Hadeed and Dr. Humberto Rey, beginning in 1983, has found that parents may hold the key to helping their premature babies. Their studies, confirmed by others, discovered the value of skin-to-skin contact for even very tiny babies.

The Kangaroo Care parent (both mothers and fathers can participate) carries the premature baby (wearing a diaper and usually a hat) chest-to-chest and skin-to-skin. A blanket covers the baby and holds in the warmth provided by the parent's body.

Research shows that the benefits to the baby include:

- a stable heart rate;
- more regular breathing;
- longer periods of sleep;

- better temperature;
- decreased crying;
- longer periods of alertness;
- more opportunities to breastfeed.

Parents also benefit from Kangaroo Care because the experience helps them to feel more confident and prepared for the day when baby comes home.

Kangaroo Care has succeeded with babies as small as 800 grams. IVs and monitors shouldn't interfere with Kangaroo Care. Generally, the baby needs to be stable and not on a ventilator.

Being held close to a parent in this way duplicates many of the experiences the premature baby had in the womb. It is a relaxing, safe environment for any newborn, but is even more important for the fragile premature baby

been done find absolutely no benefit to these widely used interventions.

Epidural anesthesia is often advised for every woman in premature labor. The theory is that this will relax her muscles, reduce her urge to push and make the birth gentler for the baby. There is no evidence that this can help the baby. For similar reasons, forceps are often used to deliver premature babies, with the goal of protecting the baby's head at birth. Research again does not support this. It is also very common to routinely do episiotomies on women who are giving birth to premature babies, once again with the intention of protecting the baby's head from pressure. As with the other interventions, there is no evidence that this is beneficial.

Of course, when you are worried about having a premature baby, you want to do all you can to make the birth easier for your baby.

However, these interventions all carry some risks and, since they have not been shown to be helpful, you may want to ask your doctor about avoiding them.

Caring for the Premature Baby

A premature baby needs special care from the minute it is born. You may have a neonatologist waiting in the delivery room to begin caring for the baby from the moment of birth, especially if the baby is very small.

Rebeka, who had premature triplets by Caesarean section, says, "I couldn't believe the crowd of people in the room. Each baby had a team assigned to him, and as the doctor lifted each baby out, he'd pass it on to the right person and everyone would rush into action. I only got little glimpses of them as they went by."

As previously mentioned, premature babies are at high risk of developing respiratory distress syndrome. A drug called surfactant, put into the baby's lungs shortly after birth, reduces the risk of RDS significantly. The evidence for this treatment is so good that the use of surfactant can be recommended routinely in the care of all very premature infants.

Having a premature baby can be a frightening experience. Your baby may look unbelievably tiny and fragile, and seeing her hooked up to monitors and respirators is alarming. You may not be able to touch or hold your baby right away, and even when you can, you might be afraid of hurting her because she's so small.

Most premature babies can't breastfeed right away, and you may have to pump your milk for weeks. However, your milk is valuable for your baby, and several studies have shown significant health benefits for premature babies who were given their mother's milk. And while it may be difficult to get started with breastfeeding, it is possible and well worth the effort.

At one time, it was believed that breastfeeding was more difficult for the premature baby than bottle-feeding, so these babies were given bottles first. Only after the babies were used to the bottle were the mothers allowed to try breastfeeding, and often by then the babies had a hard time learning to nurse properly at the breast. But researchers discovered that, in fact, breastfeeding is easier and less stressful for the premature baby.

Emily's son, Carl, was born at 30 weeks and weighed three pounds. She pumped milk for him and spent every day at the hospital, watching him grow slowly. "When he began to suck at the feeding tube, they told me I could try nursing him," she says. "He still looked so tiny, but he took my nipple right away. It was the most wonderful feeling! I'd breastfeed him every few hours during the day and they'd top him up by tube-feeding my expressed milk. Eventually he was getting all his milk at the

---

The Evidence About...
PREMATURE LABOR AND BIRTH

About 1 out of every 10 babies will be born prematurely—before 37 weeks of pregnancy. Fifty percent of the mothers who give birth prematurely do not have any identified risk factors.

Drugs are available that can stop premature labor, but they don't seem to improve the outcomes for the babies. Often labor starts again and the baby is still born prematurely. These drugs *can* buy some valuable time so that treatment can be given to help the baby's lungs mature or the mother can be transferred to a hospital with a neonatal intensive care unit.

The most successful treatment in premature labor is to give the mother corticosteroids. This reduces the risk of her baby developing respiratory distress syndrome by 50 percent. Treating the very premature baby with surfactant immediately after birth also significantly reduces the risk of respiratory distress syndrome.

The safest place for the very premature infant to be born is in a specialized center with a neonatal intensive care unit. Decisions about vaginal births and Caesarean delivery must be made on an individual basis.

There is no evidence that routine use of epidural anesthetic, forceps delivery, episiotomy or continuous fetal monitoring during labor produce a better outcome for the premature baby.

breast, and we started to make plans to bring him home."

Carl weighed five pounds the day he came home, nearly two months after his birth. "It was great to have him home, but it was a shock, too," Emily says. "I'd gotten used to sleeping through the night while he was in the hospital, but he'd wake up to nurse every two hours. It took a couple of days to build up my milk supply at night. But we all survived."

You and your premature baby have some challenges to face, but help is available. Ask about support groups for parents of premature babies that may be connected with your hospital. Just knowing how other parents coped can make a big difference.

29

Caesarean Section: Surgical Birth

Mary Elizabeth thinks Caesarean sections are wonderful. She knows that the one she had saved her life and that of her baby. "Towards the end of my pregnancy, I started having some bleeding from my vagina. I had an ultrasound done and the doctor discovered that my placenta was at the bottom of my uterus, right over my cervix. If I had gone into labor and my cervix had started to dilate, I could have bled to death. We scheduled a Caesarean for two weeks before my due date. I'm glad I had my baby now, rather than in the 'olden days,' when we both might have died."

Situations like the one Mary Elizabeth faced are pretty clear-cut: there was really no other choice for her and her baby except Caesarean section. There are other cases where the need for a Caesarean is definite: a baby in a sideways position that won't shift even after an attempt at external version, for example.

Most of the time, though, the reasons for Caesarean sections are less clear. In many parts of North America, about 20 to 25 per-cent of all babies are born by C-section. The rates in other parts of the world vary from about 5 percent to almost 50 percent. Looking at the international statistics from various countries about outcomes for both baby and mother, we find that when the Caesarean rate is lower than about 7 percent, there are higher complication rates for mothers and babies. But when the rate is higher than 7 percent, there is no corresponding improvement in outcomes. A country where about 7 percent of babies are delivered by C-section will see just as many healthy babies and mothers as a country where 25 percent are delivered surgically.

Why is this important? A Caesarean section, like any surgery, carries risks, and only when these risks are outweighed by the benefits should a Caesarean be done. If this surgery does not lead to healthier mothers and babies, it is unnecessary and potentially dangerous (as well as costly).

Caesarean section is more dangerous for the mother than a vaginal birth. The complica-tion rate from Caesareans for the mother is two to five times higher than with a vaginal birth. Infections in the incision, hemorrhage (severe bleeding), bladder and kidney infections and blood clots in the legs that can go to the lungs are all more frequent with Caesareans.

The rate of mothers dying from Caesareans (40 per 100,000 live births) is also higher than from vaginal births (10 to 14 per 100,000 live births). However, some, but not all, of the increase in the Caesarean death rate, is related to the complication for which it was performed in the first place.

Even when all goes well, the mother faces a longer period of recovery after a Caesarean birth than after a vaginal delivery, and may find it harder to begin caring for her baby and breastfeeding.

Caesarean section does not guarantee a good outcome for babies, as some people think. Caesarean section rates and infant mortality rates are not shown to be particularly related; hospitals with a Caesarean rate of 10 percent have the same infant mortality rate as those with a Caesarean rate of 25 percent.

There are risks to the baby, too. Caesarean babies are four times more likely than vaginal birth babies to breathe fast for a few hours after they are born. This is called *transient tachypnoea* of the newborn. This condition goes away without treatment, but it does mean that the baby needs more careful observation for the first few hours to make sure that she is improving. This fast breathing may be mistakenly interpreted as an early sign of infection, so the baby will be more likely to be treated with antibiotics. As well, Caesarean babies are slightly more likely to develop a serious breathing problem called respiratory distress syndrome, which does need treatment.

If the Caesarean benefits the mother or baby, these risks can be accepted as necessary. But if the Caesarean does not benefit mother or baby, these complications are unnecessary. North American Caesarean rates are considerably higher than 7 percent, and that strongly suggests that some of these Caesareans do not benefit mother or baby.

The tough question is: *Which Caesareans are unnecessary?* There are some definite answers to that, and there are still some gray areas. The next section looks at some factors that contribute to high Caesarean rates.

Why So Many Caesareans?

Previous Caesarean

At one time, the motto was "once a Caesarean, always a Caesarean"; a mother who had one Caesarean birth was told that any subsequent babies would require surgical delivery as well. Good research has clearly demonstrated that in most cases these mothers are quite capable of giving birth vaginally. Routine repeat Caesareans, done just because the mother had a previous C-section, will lead to a large number of unnecessary operations. (See Chapter 30, Vaginal Birth after Caesarean Section.)

Failure to Progress

The diagnosis of *dystocia* or "failure to progress in labor" often leads to Caesarean section. Dystocia is a general word meaning abnormal labor—doctors almost always use it to refer to labor that is progressing very slowly. The Society for Obstetricians and Gynaecologists of Canada (SOGC) has published guidelines to try to prevent labors from receiving this label too quickly, with the goal of avoiding unnecessary Caesareans. Their advice is as follows:

- A woman should not be said to be "in *active* labor" unless her cervix is 3 to 4 cm (1.2 to 1.6 in) dilated and at least 80 percent effaced. Contractions, of course, may have begun many hours or even days before this point is reached. Until the cervix has effaced and dilated to this point, the mother is considered to be in early or latent labor. Latent labor can be very long but still be normal.

- Once active labor is underway, labor needs to be observed for at least four hours to see if progress is being made. A diagnosis of dystocia can be *considered* when less than 0.5 cm (0.2 in) of dilation per hour occurs over a four-hour period.
- If labor is progressing slowly but mother and baby are both doing well, no treatment may be needed. The mother can be encouraged to walk and she should have a support person with her at all times. Before considering a Caesarean section, rupturing the membranes or using oxytocin to speed up the contractions should be tried. If the mother is exhausted and in a lot of pain, an epidural might help.

Using these SOGC guidelines for diagnosing and treating dystocia has been shown to reduce the number of Caesarean sections done for this reason, with equally good outcomes for the babies.

After 10 hours of strong contractions, Picku and her husband drove to the hospital. To Picku's surprise, the nurse told her she wasn't in active labor. "All those contractions," Picku says, "and I wasn't even 2 cm (0.8 in) dilated. I thought something was definitely wrong, but the nurse said it was normal for this stage to go slowly. They sent us home, and we went back about 12 hours later. By then I was about 5 cm (2 in) dilated, and things started moving after that."

It was only afterwards that Picku's doctor explained the guidelines to her, and then she was pleased that the nurse had sent her home.

"I was disappointed at the time, because we were so excited about being in labor. It's discouraging to be sent home again, but in reality I was more relaxed at home. And I'm glad I didn't end up with a Caesarean just because my labor started out so slowly."

Non-reassuring Fetal Heart Patterns (Fetal Distress)

Fetal distress is diagnosed when the baby shows signs of not getting enough oxygen or otherwise having trouble coping with labor, and is another common reason for Caesarean delivery.

Using an electronic fetal monitor to continuously monitor the heart rates of babies during labor definitely has been found to increase the rate of Caesarean section without improving the outcome for the babies. That means that some of the babies who were continuously monitored were delivered by Caesarean unnecessarily. Unfortunately, we don't know which ones. At present, research is trying to clarify which fetal heart rate patterns truly indicate fetal distress. To date, all the patterns identified as "non-reassuring" still include many babies who are doing well.

The best recommendation to reduce unnecessary Caesarean sections for fetal distress seems to be: don't use continuous monitoring during labor for normal pregnancies.

Labor Interventions

While research studies usually try to measure the effects of each intervention separately, in real life the interventions often are interconnected, with one leading to another. It can be difficult to tell whether a single intervention or a whole series actually led to the situation that required a Caesarean.

Consider Terry's experience, for example. Three days after her due date, she started having contractions in the middle of the night. "They were very irregular and short, lasting about 30 seconds each. I thought I probably had a long way to go, but I called my doctor anyway to let her know that I thought labor had started. The contractions continued pretty much the same way all day and through the next night, and I was tired from not sleeping very much. I went for my regular doctor's appointment, and after more than 24 hours of contractions, I was only 1 cm (0.4 in) dilated. My doctor called it 'failure to progress.'"

The kind of long latent phase of labor that Terry experienced is common. It isn't unusual for women to go through days of short, irregular contractions without the cervix dilating very much. Sometimes the labor will stop altogether and then start again at a later date. In most cases, labor will gradually or suddenly get stronger without any intervention.

Terry's doctor, however, recommended that she go to the hospital to have her labor augmented. She was put in bed, given Pitocin by IV, attached to a fetal monitor and shortly after that given an epidural. Four hours after this process was begun, Terry's doctor ruptured her membranes. At this point the baby's heart rate began to show some episodes of slowing during contractions. The Pitocin level was turned up higher. "I remember my doctor saying she wanted to get this baby born before suppertime," Terry says.

The baby's heartbeat on the fetal monitor then became more erratic, and Terry's doctor told her that the baby was in distress and a Caesarean would be necessary at once. "All I could think was that I was willing to do whatever was needed to have a healthy baby." Terry developed a fever and infection after the Caesarean and wasn't able to care for her new son (who was fine) for two days.

It's hard to second-guess a mother's birth experience, but Terry's story does show how different interventions are often related. Because she agreed to the augmentation of her labor (even though research shows that the slow latent phase she was experiencing is quite normal), her labor became more painful. (Eighty percent of women who have their labor induced or strengthened by oxytocin feel that it increases the amount of pain they experience and find it unpleasant.) She then decided on an epidural to help with the pain.

Did her natural, slowly progressing labor lead to Terry's Caesarean section, or was it the combination of the induction, fetal monitoring, restriction to bed and epidural anesthetic? Would the results have been different if her doctor had encouraged her to rest and wait at home until her contractions became stronger and more regular, or suggested walking to make the contractions more effective?

Since many interventions carry an increased risk of Caesarean section, one of the best things a woman in labor can do to minimize her risk of C-section is to avoid interventions as much as possible.

Planned Caesarean Section

If a Caesarean is recommended before labor even begins (for example, because your baby is in a breech position, or because you had a previous Caesarean section, or because your baby is "too big"), you can ask for a second opinion, just as you can for any major operation.

The Physician's Fear of Lawsuits

Half of the lawsuits filed against doctors practicing obstetrics claim that a Caesarean section should have been done to avoid whatever damage the baby suffered during delivery. These claims are made despite the complete lack of evidence that Caesarean delivery reduces childhood neurological problems, cerebral palsy or seizures.

Even when the doctor is found not to be at

Avoiding Unnecessary Caesareans

Some things you can do to help prevent a Caesarean section:

- Arrange for a doula or other trained labor support person.
- Walk around as much as possible during labor.
- Avoid routine continuous electronic fetal monitoring.
- Avoid induction unless medically indicated
- Use alternate methods of pain relief rather than an epidural; delay having an epidural for as long as possible.
- If you've had a previous Caesarean section, plan to have your next baby vaginally.
- If your baby is breech or transverse, ask to have an external version after 37 weeks.

fault, dealing with a lawsuit is expensive, time-consuming and stressful.

It is impossible to quantify how much the fear of being sued affects doctors' decision making about doing Caesareans. However, as one example, although the research shows that careful forceps deliveries are just as safe as Caesarean sections, the rate of forceps deliveries has decreased and the rate of Caesarean sections has increased. Doctors feel that if something does go wrong, they are less likely to be sued if it happens after a Caesarean section rather than after a forceps delivery.

Since "the fear of being sued" is impossible to measure or research, hard data on this are not available. However, it is definitely an issue for doctors today.

When a Caesarean Is Required

Anesthetic

You and your doctor have decided that a Caesarean is required to safely deliver your baby. This decision may have been made before labor, because of the baby's position, placenta previa or other complications, or it may have been made during labor because the baby is in distress or the umbilical cord has prolapsed, for example, or it may have been made at the end of labor when attempts to deliver the baby with forceps have failed or there are other problems. Just as for any other surgery, you will need to have anesthetic to stop you from feeling the pain.

Modern anesthetic techniques, with special modifications for pregnancy, make anesthesia during Caesarean section extremely safe for both mother and baby. To try to put it in perspective, the risk of the mother dying from having a baby (by Caesarean or not) is between 10 and 14 per 100,000 live births. Anesthesia complications will cause only one of these deaths—a very low number.

For Caesareans, the most common type of anesthetic is regional—usually an epidural or a spinal. Mothers usually like the idea of being awake to see the baby as soon as it is born. Sometimes mothers are interested in being awake, but are worried about seeing the surgery. You might be reassured to know that a drape will be hung over your chest so that you won't see any of the gory parts. With regional anesthesia, you often will feel touch and pressure during the surgery. If you feel pain, the anesthetist can give you more painkillers or a general anesthetic.

Regional anesthetics avoid the risk of the mother vomiting while she is unconscious. The biggest concern with these regional anesthetics is that the mother's blood pressure will drop, so she is given extra fluids through an IV before the surgery.

A general anesthetic, which makes the mother unconscious during the operation, may be a better choice in a few situations. Mothers with bleeding problems are likely to have more serious complications if they have an epidural, so a general anesthetic would be recommended. A general anesthetic can also be given more quickly than an epidural, so it's the best choice when speed is critical. The biggest risk of general anesthetic is aspiration pneumonia. Giving antacids immediately before putting the mother to sleep cuts down on the risk of severe aspiration pneumonia.

Many women who have an epidural or spinal anesthetic during a Caesarean want to have their partners or support people with them. The experience of surgery is pretty stressful, and having that emotional support can make a big difference. Your partner can hold the baby once he is born and bring him to you so you can touch him and have a good look. Most hospitals now permit at least one support person during Caesareans, but a few still restrict them to planned and pre-scheduled Caesareans only.

Some mothers also want their partners there even if they have a general anesthetic. The partner will be able to tell the mother afterwards what happened, and will be able to hold the baby. However, most hospitals discourage or forbid the partner's presence when the mother is having a general anesthetic.

Step by Step through a Caesarean

Once the decision is made to deliver the baby by Caesarean section, an intravenous will be started, a catheter will be put in your bladder to drain urine and the top part of your pubic hair will be shaved.

You will be moved to an operating room (usually in the labor and delivery department, but occasionally in another part of the hospital). This room is brightly lit, stocked with sur-

Meet the Team

Once the decision has been made to do a Caesarean section, a team of people gather together for the surgery.

The obstetrician is the surgeon who will actually do the Caesarean. This may be the person who cared for you during your pregnancy, or another doctor who has been called in. A second doctor will be involved to assist–this might be a resident or your family doctor, if available.

If your family doctor cared for you during pregnancy, he or she will have called in the obstetrician to consult on the problem that made the Caesarean necessary. Your family doctor may assist during the operation.

An anesthetist will give you either a general anesthetic (putting you to sleep) or a regional anesthetic (freezing you from the waist down). He or she will talk to you during the process and explain what is happening.

A pediatrician or nursery nurse with special training will take care of the baby from birth.

Two nurses will help with the surgery by passing the doctors the needed instruments and equipment.

Your partner has an important job, too–holding your hand, telling you what's happening and greeting your baby as she is born.

gical instruments and sterile gowns and has a table with a heater over it for the baby. During your surgery, all the medical personnel will wear gowns, hats and face masks.

If you are having a spinal or epidural, the anesthetist will put it in now. Then your abdomen will be washed with soap and you will

Caesarean Incisions

The incision in the skin is most often transverse (from side to side) just at the top of your pubic hair. This is sometimes called a bikini cut, because it won't show if you wear a bikini. The skin incision may also be vertical, going from just below the belly button to the top of the pubic hair.

The incision in the uterus is almost always transverse across the bottom of the uterus. This incision is stronger when it heals and safer during the next pregnancy. In rare cases, because of the position of the baby or the placenta, a vertical incision must be used. In a few cases, the doctor starts off by doing a transverse incision, but has to add a vertical one to get the baby out. Then the mother has a scar like an upside-down T on her uterus.

The direction of the skin incision has nothing to do with the direction of the incision in the uterus. They may be the same or different. A transverse incision on the uterus is definitely preferable, because it will be stronger during subsequent pregnancies and births.

be covered with clean sheets, leaving a gap in the middle for your belly. If you are having a general anesthetic, the sheets will be put in place first, then the anesthetist will put you to sleep (this is done at the last minute so the baby gets as little anesthesia as possible). Sheets are pinned up on poles by your chest so that if you are awake you won't see the actual surgery.

The first cut goes through the skin and fat down to the muscle. Then the abdominal muscles are pulled apart and cut to get to the peritoneum. This is cut, too, and right underneath it is the uterus, filling the whole abdomen.

Another incision is made in the uterus—some amniotic fluid will gush out at this point—and the baby is pulled out through the incision, the umbilical cord is clamped and cut and the baby is immediately handed to the pediatrician. Then the placenta is pulled out through the incision. This whole part—from giving the anesthetic to delivering the baby—takes about 10 minutes.

The baby is out, but now the doctor has to stitch you back together. First, the incision in the uterus has to be carefully sewed up in layers. Then the peritoneum is closed up. The muscle layer is tacked back together, and the skin is closed with stitches, staples or tiny bandages called steristrips. This part of the birth takes 30 to 45 minutes.

If you have had a general, the anesthetic will be stopped at this point and you will start to wake up. If you have had a regional anesthetic, you have probably been admiring your new baby. You will now move to a recovery room, where a nurse will make frequent checks of your breathing and blood pressure. Usually the catheter in your bladder is left in for several hours, and the IV is left in for a day or two.

Alex remembers: "They rushed Shirley into the operating room for the Caesarean and told me I'd have to wait outside because they were giving her a general. It seemed like just a couple of minutes when the nurse came out with my baby girl. I picked her up for a second and admired her, and then the nurse took her away to be weighed and everything. I stood there waiting for Shirley to come out, and I didn't know why it was taking so long. Nobody told me that it was normal. I was convinced that something terrible had happened to her and began trying to figure out how I'd cope as a single father. It was more than 45 minutes before they wheeled Shirley out, and I was so relieved to find out she was okay."

Recovering from a Caesarean Section

- You have had major surgery, so expect your recovery to be slower than if you'd had a vaginal birth.
- About one in five women will have a fever and infection; antibiotics given at the time of the surgery reduce this.
- You may have gas pains and be constipated. Eat lightly for the first two days, and walk around as much as possible.
- You will have a catheter in your bladder for several hours at least. It may be difficult and uncomfortable to urinate at first when the catheter comes out.
- You will probably have an IV for a day or two, to provide fluids and pain medication.
- You will feel pain at the incision site–some women say it feels like their insides are falling out! It can help to press your hands or a small pillow against the incision when you get up or walk around.
- It can be a challenge to find a comfortable position for breastfeeding. Put a pillow under the baby to protect the incision, or ask your nurse or a lactation consultant to show you how to nurse on your side or using a football hold.
- Your emotional reactions may be quite intense. Some women are extremely disappointed about having a Caesarean, even when they know it was necessary. Ask your caregivers about support groups in your community; it often helps to talk to other new mothers about your feelings.

Recovery

After the surgery is over, the mother faces a recovery period just as she would after any operation. One common complication from Caesareans is infection, and about one in five mothers will have a fever and other signs of infection during the first few days after they have given birth; some of these mothers will be seriously ill. The risk of infection is higher for women who have been in labor for some time before the surgery, for those whose membranes ruptured before the surgery and for obese women.

Because post-Caesarean infections are so common, they have been studied carefully. The research has now clearly established that giving antibiotics to the mother at the time of the Caesarean will significantly reduce the rate of infection. This is most often done through the IV after the baby is born and the umbilical cord has been clamped, so the drug isn't passed on to the baby.

Jennifer's advice to mothers who have Caesareans: "Make sure you have help when you get home. With the shorter hospital stays that seem to be the rule now, it's essential. When I got home I still couldn't stand up straight and walk—I'd lean my elbows on the change table to change the baby's diapers. I was so tired, I definitely needed more sleep than the baby. Remember that you've been through surgery, and get the help and rest you need."

The Evidence About . . .
CAESAREAN SECTIONS

In some situations, Caesarean sections can save the lives of mothers and babies.

However, when the rate of Caesareans is higher than about 7 percent, there is no improvement in outcomes for mothers or babies. The North American rate of 20 to 25 percent clearly puts mothers at risk without improving outcomes for babies.

Using the SOGC guidelines for VBACs and dystocia will reduce the rate of Caesarean sections. Avoiding the use of continuous monitoring will also reduce the number of Caesareans.

Giving antibiotics to the mother during the Caesarean will significantly reduce her risks of developing an infection.

30

Vaginal Birth after Caesarean Section (VBAC)

Rose's baby girl, Shannon, now four, was delivered by Caesarean section because she was in a breech position. When Rose became pregnant again, she assumed she'd plan for a second Caesarean. But one of the mothers at Shannon's day care told her she'd had a VBAC with her second pregnancy.

"What's a VBAC?" Rose asked.

"It stands for vaginal birth after Caesarean. For me, it was a million times better than having another C-section. You should talk to your doctor about it."

With her doctor's appointment several weeks away, Rose decided to do some research on her own, and discovered there was a VBAC support group in her community. The group leaders had some interesting information, and she began to wonder whether she would prefer to give birth vaginally.

For many years, obstetricians in North America have been very ready to perform a Caesarean section on all women who have had a previous Caesarean section. Generally, the mother was scheduled for her next Caesarean section between 38 and 40 weeks of pregnancy, without waiting for labor to start. This is called a booked, elective or repeat Caesarean section. If labor started before the scheduled date, the mother was instructed to come to the hospital immediately, and a Caesarean section would be performed at once without waiting to see if labor would progress.

Doctors planned these repeat Caesareans because they believed that to have a second surgical delivery was safer than the mother going into labor and trying to give birth vaginally. They were concerned that the scar on her uterus might rupture. They also assumed that most women who have had a Caesarean section would wind up needing one again with their next labor. Both of these assumptions have been shown to be false.

Initially, it wasn't physicians who doubted these assumptions. While many women with Caesareans accepted the advice they were given and arranged for repeat C-sections, some women decided to try giving birth vaginally. At first, there were no studies and few statistics to support their choices. It was often difficult to find a doctor willing to attend a VBAC birth, and many hospitals set up procedures that made it difficult. Women persisted, though—sometimes by deciding to have a VBAC at home—and gradually the statistics accumulated.

Randomized controlled studies have not been performed to compare the outcome of elective Caesarean section with a "trial of labor" (the mother going into labor and only having a Caesarean for the usual reasons), because women will not agree to be randomly assigned to Caesarean section or labor. The information we have comes from studying two large groups of similar women. One group had trials of labor after Caesarean section; the other group had elective repeat Caesarean section. Researchers found two important results:

- Trial of labor after Caesarean section (with a transverse lower uterine segment incision) is safer for the mother and as safe for the baby as repeat elective Caesarean section.
- With trial of labor, almost 80 percent of women deliver vaginally.

The biggest concern that has been raised about having a VBAC is that there may be a risk of uterine rupture. This does not mean that the uterus explodes; it means that the scar from the previous Caesarean splits open. But this is very serious. It causes immediate pain, shock, internal bleeding and fetal distress, and the baby must be delivered promptly by an emergency Caesarean section. The risk of this complication is very low, provided the previous Caesarean left a transverse lower uterine segment incision. What's a "transverse lower uterine segment incision"? For the past 40 years,

the vast majority of Caesarean sections have been done with this kind of cut. It means that the obstetrician has cut sideways across the bottom of the uterus (the lower uterine segment), which isn't very muscular and does not contract during labor.

The older, "classical" incision is cut vertically in the uterus and goes through the more muscular upper part of the uterus, which does contract during labor. Currently, this kind of incision is used very rarely. Occasionally, an "inverted T" incision may be used, in which first a transverse lower uterine incision is made, and then, if there is difficulty getting the baby out (as can happen with a breech position), the doctor creates extra room by adding a vertical incision up through the lower uterine segment and into the muscular upper segment. The appearance of the skin incision—up and down or across the abdomen—has nothing to do with the uterine incision.

With a transverse lower uterine incision, the chance of rupture of the uterus is very small—the risk is from 0.09 to 0.22 percent.

There are very little data on women who have labored after having a classical incision in their upper uterine segment. Best estimates of the risk of rupture range from 2.2 percent to 14 percent. Data on women laboring with an inverted T incision are also limited: the current best estimate suggests a risk of rupture of about 1.3 percent.

Rupture with a vertical incision is not only more likely than with a transverse lower segment incision, it is much more dangerous for the baby. The baby is more likely to be expelled from the uterus into the abdominal cavity, and there is more likely to be significant separation of the placenta. This rupture is just as likely to occur before the onset of labor as it is during labor, making it difficult to prevent by elective Caesarean section unless surgery is performed well before term.

Other Safety Considerations

There are other complications, besides the rather dramatic one of uterine rupture, to be considered in comparing VBACs and repeat Caesareans.

Very few women die having babies, but more women die having Caesarean sections than having vaginal births. Because some of these deaths are from the conditions that prompted the Caesarean (such as severe pre-eclampsia) and not the surgery itself, it is difficult to estimate the actual risk from Caesarean section. When researchers sift out other factors, they conclude that the risk of a mother dying from an elective Caesarean section is two to four times the risk of dying from a vaginal birth.

Mothers having Caesarean sections are more likely to develop wound infections, pneumonia, bleeding requiring blood transfusion, urinary tract infections and uterine infections. These are all lumped together and called "morbidity." The morbidity rate is higher among women who have elective repeat C-sections than among those who have a trial of labor—and the trial of labor group includes both those who deliver vaginally and those who end up having a second Caesarean section. It's clear from these statistics that a planned VBAC is safer than a repeat Caesarean section for the mother.

What about the safety of the baby? The death rates and complication rates for the babies are the same for both groups in the studies that report these data.

The main risk of Caesarean delivery for the baby is that it will develop either a fast breathing rate, called transient tachypnoea, or a more serious breathing problem, called respiratory distress syndrome, in the first few hours after birth. Both transient tachypnoea and respiratory distress syndrome are more common after Caesarean section than after vaginal

Politics, Dollars and VBACs

Economically, VBAC is an idea whose time has come. It is much less expensive for the health care system to do a vaginal birth than a Caesarean. The evidence that it is also safer has been great news for the organizations that pay for health care.

Some U.S. health insurers are suggesting that a trial of labor after a previous Caesarean section will be paid for, but an elective repeat Caesarean may not be.

birth. Since 80 percent of the babies whose mothers choose to have a trial of labor will be born vaginally, this reduces their risk of both conditions.

Also, there is always a risk of doing the elective Caesarean prematurely as a result of mistaken dates or inaccurate ultrasound estimates.

Thinking about VBAC

What should Rose consider as she plans the birth of her second baby?

First, she needs to know what kind of incision she has in her uterus. The risk of uterine rupture is about 0.1 to 0.2 percent with a lower uterine segment transverse incision, about 1.3 percent with an inverted T incision and 2.2 to 14 percent with a classical incision vertically in the upper uterine segment.

Rose doesn't need to think too much about the reason for her first Caesarean. The reason for the previous Caesarean section makes only a marginal difference in the success rate of VBAC. Researchers originally thought that some reasons for Caesarean section—such as labor that stops progressing, or a baby too big to fit through the pelvis—were more likely to recur and require a second Caesarean than complications such as a breech presentation. But this theory has not proved true. Even with a previous diagnosis of abnormal labor causing the first C-section, 75 percent of women were able to deliver vaginally during a trial of labor. Many women have vaginally delivered bigger babies than the one for which they had a Caesarean.

Rose has had only one previous Caesarean delivery, but some women have had two or three before planning a VBAC. The studies to date, although small, do not suggest any significant differences in success rate or complication rate for women who have a trial of labor after more than one Caesarean section.

A previous vaginal delivery as well as the previous Caesarean does increase the chances of a successful trial of labor. Diane, for example, had two normal vaginal births. When she went into labor with her third baby, he was in a transverse position—lying sideways—and was delivered by Caesarean section. With her fourth pregnancy, she confidently planned a VBAC. "I knew I could have a baby vaginally," Diane says. "I'd done it twice. So having a VBAC didn't seem like a big deal to me."

For Rose and other women contemplating a VBAC, there are often emotional issues as well. Hanna was in labor for more than 30 hours before she had a Caesarean because her baby was in distress. She vividly remembers how painful and exhausting her long labor was, and how scared she felt at the end when they rushed her into the operating room. It's an experience she won't risk repeating; she plans to have an elective repeat C-section with her next baby.

Iris also had a long and difficult labor before her surgery, and she was very disappointed when it ended up in a Caesarean. When she became pregnant again, she decided to plan for a VBAC. But it wasn't easy making that choice.

"I had so many conflicting feelings," Iris says. "I really didn't want another Caesarean, but I was terrified of another long, hard labor. And what if I went through it again and then had another Caesarean after all? Even with support from the VBAC group I belonged to, I felt pretty anxious about the whole thing."

Knowing that labor is safe after a Caesarean doesn't always balance out the mother's fears of having to go through a painful experience that might end up, once again, in surgery. If the Caesarean was done partway through their first labor, women wonder just how much worse it can get. Will they be able to cope with the end of labor and pushing out a baby? First-time mothers wonder about these questions, too, but the Caesarean mother often feels like her body didn't work properly the first time, and might fail her again.

As Iris found out, support groups for VBAC mothers can help work through those fears. Other women have found information and support by reading books such as *Silent Knife* by Nancy Wainer Cohen or by contacting others on the Internet.

The VBAC Labor

When mothers decide to have a VBAC, should their labors be handled differently than "normal" labors? *The combined conclusion of many research studies is that women who have had a Caesarean section, and who go into labor with a later pregnancy, should be treated no differently than any other laboring women.*

The use of oxytocin to induce or speed up labor has not increased the rate of uterine rupture, although this may just reflect the fact that the trials have been small and rupture is a rare complication. At present, it seems reasonable to recommend that oxytocin drugs be used with the same care that should attend their use

A Difficult Decision: Ann's VBAC

For some women, the VBAC decision is readily supported. For others, it is more challenging.

Ann's first baby was in a breech position. When her labor seemed to be progressing very slowly, her doctor became concerned and strongly recommended a Caesarean. During the surgery, he had trouble getting the baby out. He initially made a transverse incision across the bottom of Ann's uterus; now he added a vertical one so that the whole incision looked like an upside-down T on her uterus.

Before Ann left the hospital, the obstetrician met with her and explained how the surgery had gone. "If you have another baby, it will have to be delivered by Caesarean because of that incision," he told her.

Ann recalls: "I didn't get pregnant again for four years because I couldn't bear the idea of another C-section. I still feel that I didn't need that first Caesarean; I just let myself get talked into it."

When she did conceive again, Ann was determined to have a VBAC. But it turned out to be much harder than she had expected. "I went to see eight different doctors. As soon as they heard about my incision, they stopped talking to me. They all said I had to have a Caesarean and that was that. One doctor told me I had a 50 percent risk of my uterus rupturing and me and the baby dying. Most of the others just said it was unacceptable."

Ann felt strongly that she was not being irrational or unreasonable. She had carefully researched her situation. Since incisions like hers are rare, she did not have a lot to go on, but the rate of uterine rupture seems to be between 1 and 2 percent. This is certainly higher than the risks of a repeat Caesarean, but Ann felt the risk was acceptable to her.

The ninth doctor Ann spoke to agreed to provide her care during this pregnancy. They discussed the risks and the doctor reminded Ann that the choice she was making was not the safest route.

But it was Ann's choice. As she points out, "We know that the safest choice for a woman with a lower transverse incision is to have a VBAC, yet many women choose to have a repeat Caesarean. It's not the safest choice, but those women rarely have any problems finding a doctor who is prepared to do another C-section for them."

By then, Ann was 32 weeks. The rest of her pregnancy went smoothly—her baby was head-down and average in size. When labor started, Ann and her husband went to the hospital right away. Ann had a five-hour labor (most of it spent in the shower) and a straightforward delivery of a lovely little girl.

It's not surprising that Ann gave birth to a healthy baby vaginally, despite having an "inverted T" incision. The statistics tell us that between 98 and 99 percent of the women in her situation will do exactly that.

What's significant about Ann's story is that she made her own decision, despite running up against some opposition. She understood the research, assessed the risks and made a responsible choice. Even if she had experienced a complication because of her incision, it would not have changed the validity of her decision-making process.

The Evidence About...
VBAC

A woman who has had a previous Caesarean section with a lower uterine segment incision should be encouraged to have a trial of labor with her next pregnancy. National consensus statements in Canada and the United States recommend trial of labor.

The likelihood of a successful vaginal birth is not significantly changed by the reason for the first Caesarean section or the number of previous Caesarean sections.

Care in labor is the same as should be offered to any laboring woman. The hospital facilities, monitoring of the baby, the use of oxytocin induction or stimulation of labor and epidural anesthesia may be used for the same reasons as for any woman in labor.

The woman who is considering a trial of labor after a Caesarean section in which a classical incision was performed has a higher risk of uterine rupture and increased risk over elective Caesarean section.

caregivers will know if the scar on her uterus ruptures because the baby will show signs of distress.

Until recently, a doctor would sometimes insert his hand through the vagina and cervix after a VBAC birth to feel the inside of the uterus and check for any problems with the scar. Studies have shown that this is not helpful: it is very painful for the mother (unless she has had an epidural), there is an increased risk of infection and it usually gives little helpful information. It's more important to watch the mother for excessive bleeding after the baby is born.

Having their babies in "high-risk" or teaching hospitals rather than in community hospitals does not improve outcomes to mothers having VBACs. Some women may choose to have VBACs at home.

Monica says, "When I was pregnant with Eric (after having a Caesarean with her first baby, Adam), the doctor told me I had to come to the hospital as soon as I had a contraction to be hooked up to an IV and a fetal monitor. I was told I couldn't have any painkillers so that I'd notice right away if my uterus ruptured. I don't know anything that makes it harder to relax during contractions than trying to feel if your uterus is rupturing! My labor took quite a while, but I did manage to give birth vaginally."

When Monica conceived again, she read more about how VBAC labors should be treated. "This time I decided to labor at home most of the time, where I was more comfortable and relaxed. I was only at the hospital for two hours—with no IV or monitor—when the baby was born."

in any labor. Some hospitals suggest that if oxytocin is being used in a VBAC labor, an obstetrician and anesthetist should be immediately available.

Women in VBAC labors can have epidurals if they want, without increased risk. Although the mother doesn't feel pain, her

Part Six

Your Baby's First 48 Hours

Adrienne Leong

Once upon a time, new mothers stayed in the hospital for five to seven days. That's rarely the case these days—most women go home between 24 and 48 hours after their babies are born. During that short period of time you have lots to learn about your baby and about becoming a mother.

You may have decided to give birth at home. You will be learning the basics of baby care in your own bedroom, perhaps with the help of your midwife or doula.

One of the biggest challenges for many new mothers is learning how to breastfeed. Those first few days can be very important in getting the breastfeeding relationship underway and preventing future problems.

To get you and your baby off to the best start, here's the best evidence on caring for a newborn and establishing breastfeeding.

31

You and Your Newborn Baby

How can you best welcome your newborn baby into the world? Certainly, like any human being, your new baby should be treated with gentleness and respect. The choice of how to demonstrate that loving welcome is up to you.

Dr. Frederick Leboyer emphasized gentleness in handling the newborn, to reduce the trauma of the baby's sudden separation from his mother into a loud, noisy, bright room. He recommended a dim delivery room, delayed clamping of the umbilical cord, silence except for the parents' voices, gentle massage and a warm bath for the infant. Small studies of all of these measures have not shown any specific effect on the newborn's health, good or bad. You should think about what appeals to you and makes sense to you, and ask for those things to be done.

Meeting Your Baby

Most new mothers want to touch and hold their babies as soon as possible. It seems to be a biological process. Petra remembers reaching out for her newborn baby, only to be told that the doctor had to finish stitching her up first. The baby was placed in a bassinet with plastic sides and a radiant heater overhead, and Petra remembers tears running down her cheeks as she looked longingly at her baby. "I just wanted to touch him," she says.

Fathers may have mixed feelings. Some are eager to hold their newly born babies; others feel suddenly apprehensive. Tarik remembers the nurse wrapping the baby in a towel and saying, "Here you go, Dad." He says, "It was like my arms were paralyzed. I was afraid I might drop him or make him cry or do something wrong. He was so small and I felt so awkward. I'd never even seen a baby that tiny before."

But Rob felt quite differently. When his wife, Sheila, had a Caesarean, "As soon as Miranda was born, the nurse wrapped her up and handed her to me. I held her close to Sheila's face so she could see her, and then unwrapped her a little so we could both check that she had all her fingers and toes. I liked being the first one to hold her."

"Are Babies Supposed to Look Like That?"

If you haven't seen many brand-new babies, you may be surprised by your newborn's appearance.

- Baby's head may be elongated or cone-shaped. This is called molding and it will go away in a few days.
- Baby's face may be puffy and her eyes may not open much at first.
- The baby's eyes may cross from time to time.
- There may be bruises or marks from the forceps or vacuum extractor.
- The soft spot on the top of baby's head may seem quite large and it will pulsate.
- Babies are often born coated with a white, creamy substance called vernix.
- Baby may have dark hair on his back and shoulders, called lanugo. It will disappear in a few weeks.
- The baby's genitals may look swollen. Baby girls sometimes have some bleeding from the vagina.

Norah's midwife urged her to touch her baby's head as it emerged from her vagina, and she reached down to feel the hair. "It felt so weird," she says, "but it made it seem real. As he was born my midwife said, 'Take him, take him,' and I pulled him up onto my chest and it was wonderful." The surge of emotion she felt as she held her wet baby against her skin is still vivid and intense in her memory.

Mothers are sometimes surprised by the intensity of their feelings once the baby is born. Sandra knew her hospital's policy was to keep all babies in the nursery for eight hours after birth for observation, and she thought it

sounded like a reasonable idea. Her doctor explained to her that she would be too tired after labor and giving birth to look after the baby, anyway. But when Sandra's son was born, she found she couldn't bear the thought of being separated from him. When he was taken off to the nursery, she was too restless and anxious to sleep—she wanted him with her. Finally she got out of bed and walked down to the nursery hoping to at least see her baby. When she arrived, she was upset to find that he was crying in his bassinet and nobody was paying any attention. A nurse escorted her back to her room, where she tossed and turned until her baby was finally brought to her. When Sandra's second baby was born, she let the hospital know in advance that the baby was to stay with her from birth.

Not all mothers feel that way. Cheryl was very tired after a long, hard labor and somewhat groggy from pain medication. She says, "I expected to be all excited once the baby was born. Instead, I felt distant. I was just glad it was over, and I wanted to go to sleep."

Anne says, "I remember looking at my daughter and saying, 'Hello, stranger.' I knew she was my baby, but I didn't feel any connection to her. It took me a while to get to know her and fall in love with her."

If the mother is tired or experiencing the side-effects of pain medication, the hospital staff may suggest taking the baby to the nursery. The baby's father might choose to hold the baby and keep the new family together, or he might follow the baby to the nursery and supervise the process of weighing, examining and bathing the baby.

Keeping mother and baby together after birth is important, not just because mothers prefer it, but because it produces better outcomes for mothers and babies. One well-conducted study found that the risk of child abuse and neglect was lower when mothers and babies "roomed-in" together from birth, compared to mothers and babies who were separated for most of their hospital stay.

Other studies have noted more affectionate behavior and more self-confidence when mothers kept their babies with them. Mothers who kept their babies with them are also more likely to succeed at breastfeeding, and to breastfeed for longer than three months.

Researchers have observed typical ways in which many mothers greet and examine their new babies. A mother will often study her baby's face without saying much until the baby opens his eyes, and then she will speak softly to the baby, saying "hello" or "there you are" or calling the baby by name. She will touch the baby first with the tips of her fingers and then with her whole hand, and will usually undress the baby (if she has been wrapped in a blanket or gown) and examine the baby's entire body. The freedom to go through this process in her own way, and at her own speed, seems to be important for the new mother as she builds a connection with her baby.

All of this does not mean that mothers and babies who miss that immediate "bonding" time because of hospital routines, illness or other complications will have problems relating or will never fall in love with each other. They will! But the hours immediately after birth do seem to be a sensitive time, when both mother and baby are primed to make that connection. Caregivers and hospitals should promote this time together, and not infringe on it with unnecessary routines.

Fathers and new babies have not been studied in the same way as mothers and babies have been.

The risk of the baby catching an infection while in the hospital is significant, and any infection can be serious in a newborn infant. At least one study found lower rates of infection in babies who roomed-in with their mothers when compared to babies who stayed in the nursery. Hospital routines to prevent infection, including using gowns and restricting visitors, have not been demonstrated to reduce infection rates.

Routine Treatments of the Newborn

Will keeping the mother and baby together interfere with the care the baby receives? What immediate care do healthy newborns need?

The doctor, nurse or midwife will usually suction the baby's mouth and nose as soon as it is born. This hasn't been studied, even though it is so frequently done. It is intended to clear any mucus or fluid from the baby's airway so that he can breathe more easily. There are some risks: if it is done too vigorously, the baby can bleed from her mouth or nose, or the catheter can cause spasms in the baby's throat and abnormal heartbeats.

If the baby has passed meconium before birth, suctioning of the nose, mouth and throat as soon as the baby's head emerges may help to prevent the baby inhaling any meconium into his lungs. This procedure is safe enough to be recommended, although its benefit has never been demonstrated in clinical trials.

"I wish somebody had told me beforehand that they always suction babies," Mieke says. "When the doctor yelled at the nurse, 'Okay, suction here,' I panicked. I thought something must be wrong. And the baby made this horrible gurgling and gagging noise that scared me even more. But the doctor and nurse were completely calm and unconcerned, so I realized everything was okay. Then Theo started to cry, and it was the most beautiful sound I had ever heard."

The other concern is to keep the baby warm. Even healthy newborns can lose a lot of heat in a cold room (and many hospital delivery rooms are air-conditioned), and infants cool down even more quickly because they are wet at birth. The best way to keep your baby warm is to gently dry her with a warm towel, then settle her, tummy-down, against your bare chest. The two of you can then be covered with a prewarmed blanket, or a heater could be set up near you if necessary. The newborn examination can be done while the baby is in your arms or lying beside you (roll over onto your side so that you can see her better).

If the mother is unable to hold the baby, the baby can be wrapped well and given to the father to hold, or can be placed in a bassinet with a heater overhead for warmth. The father could also remove his shirt and have the baby against his bare skin with a blanket around the two of them.

If the baby requires resuscitation, a prewarmed area must be available so that the baby does not get cold. As much as possible should be done where the parents can still see their baby.

When Margaret's son was born, he didn't breathe well at first. The nurse moved him quickly to a heated bassinet and continued to suction him. James followed, and from his position beside the bassinet described to Margaret what was going on: "He's opened his eyes now and he's looking at me. He probably thinks I'm the one sticking that tube in his mouth. Oh—did you hear that? He sneezed. And now he's crying. His little face is all red." This running commentary was incredibly reassuring to Margaret.

Another routine treatment is swabbing the umbilical cord stump with either Neomycin or Triple dye. This has been shown to reduce the incidence of staphylococcal skin infection.

An injection of vitamin K has been given routinely to newborns to prevent "hemorrhagic disease of the newborn," a rare condition in which the baby's clotting mechanism is deficient because of lack of vitamin K. The incidence of this disease is probably 1 in 200 to 1 in 400 or less, and significant complications from the disease are much less than that.

Studies on hemorrhagic disease were done when first feedings of babies were often delayed by 12 or even 24 hours, and breastfed infants were routinely supplemented so that the infant did not get much of the colostrum (the early breast milk), which is high in vitamin K. It is probable that the risk of this disease for breastfed babies is even lower than the statistics suggest.

However, routine injections of vitamin K makes the risk even lower, and there do not seem to be any harmful effects. Vitamin K can also be given by mouth. However, new studies showing that the oral dose is not as well absorbed by the body as the injected form have prompted the Canadian Paediatric Society (CPS) to release new guidelines for the administration of vitamin K to newborns.

The CPS recommends that all newborns receive vitamin K by injection within six hours of birth. If parents choose an oral dose, the CPS recommends giving this at the first feeding, with follow-up doses during the first six to eight weeks of life. CPS cautions that parents should be aware that the oral dose is not as effective in preventing the disease as the injected dose. This is something you could discuss with your doctor if you would prefer that your baby not have the injection.

In many countries, the law requires that all newborn babies have their eyes treated to prevent gonorrhea. Silver nitrate should not be used, as it is irritating to the eyes and ineffective against infection with chlamydia. Either tetracycline or erythromycin antibiotic ointment is a better choice.

The ointment may blur the baby's vision temporarily, so the baby may not look as alertly at you. There is no urgency to put the ointment in the baby's eyes; it can be delayed until you and your baby have had a long visit, a chance to breastfeed and an opportunity to get to know each other a little.

No matter what the usual routines are at the hospital where your baby is born, understand that you have the right to refuse any treatment or procedure. You can insist on keeping your newborn with you, insist on feeding your baby whenever you (and the baby) wish, leave earlier than the hospital's normal discharge time and ask that the baby wear clothes you have brought from home rather than the hospital's gowns.

Establishing "family-centered maternity care" is a goal of most hospitals and is encouraged by guidelines published by both the Canadian and American colleges of obstetricians and gynecologists. Institutes in both countries encourage hospitals to become sensitive to the needs of families. You can help this trend by letting the hospital know before you deliver what kind of care you would like. After you go home, take a minute to write to the hospital to tell them all the things you liked (or didn't like) about your stay. It makes a difference!

32

Getting Started with Breastfeeding

Why Choose Breastfeeding?

Annette says: "I decided to breastfeed because of the allergies in both my family and my husband's family. I've really suffered with mine, and I wanted to prevent them if I could."

Noor says: "Breastfeeding just seemed like the normal thing to do. You know—human milk for human babies, cow's milk for calves..."

Rena says: "Shaila will be in daycare soon, and I think that because I'm breastfeeding her she won't be sick as often. That means not only is she happier and healthier, but I have less time off from work."

Celine says: "When I started really looking at the benefits of breastfeeding, I was amazed. It really does make a difference in so many areas. I want my baby to have the best possible start, and I know that means breastfeeding."

The benefits of breastfeeding have been solidly demonstrated and ongoing research continues to come up with new ones.

Knowing this, the vast majority of mothers want to breastfeed their babies; unfortunately,

Some Benefits of Breastfeeding

Breastfed babies have:

- fewer respiratory infections and fewer ear infections;
- fewer gastrointestinal infections, less diarrhea, less constipation;
- fewer and less severe allergies, including food allergies, eczema and asthma;
- lower rates of iron-deficiency anemia;
- better jaw and dental development—less likely to need braces or other orthodontic work;
- fewer admissions to hospital;
- lower incidence of SIDS (Sudden Infant Death Syndrome);
- fewer cases of a number of chronic diseases including juvenile diabetes;
- higher scores on IQ tests;
- lower rates of childhood cancers.

many of them will give up or wean early because they run into problems and don't get the help they need. What happens during labor, birth and the first few feedings can have a lot to do with the success or failure of breastfeeding.

Glenda's labor went very slowly at first, then quickly at the end. "I had been given Demerol in labor because they thought it would be several hours before the baby was born," she says. "Then suddenly things went fast and Gordon was born an hour later. Because of the Demerol, we were both pretty sleepy. I tried to nurse him but honestly, I could barely hold him, and he was out of it, too."

Glenda fell asleep, and woke up six hours later. "I asked the nurse to bring Gordon to me and she did. He had a pacifier in his mouth because they said he'd been crying a lot. I tried to nurse him then and it was pretty awkward, I don't think he really got any milk."

The next time Glenda tried to feed her son, she couldn't get him to nurse at all. "I was in tears, and Gordon was screaming. The nurse said we'd better get some food into him, and brought me a bottle of formula. He drank it right down. I guess he was starving."

Four hours later, Glenda tried again and finally got the baby to nurse. "I was so relieved. It really hurt, though, and I hadn't expected that. The nurse said some pain was normal until my nipples got toughened up."

Glenda went home with her baby boy and the hospital "new mother gift pack" that included a sample can of formula. When her nipples became even more painful a day later, she decided to give the baby another bottle of formula from the free sample, to give her nipples a break from feeding. But they hurt even more by the next day, so she gave another bottle and within a couple of weeks, Gordon was completely formula-fed.

Glenda was very disappointed that breast-feeding hadn't worked out for her, but she didn't realize that some of the problems she encountered were due to some not-very-helpful routines and policies at the hospital where her baby was born.

The Best Start

What will help breastfeeding mothers and babies get off to the best start?

Keeping mothers and babies together after birth is very helpful. When babies nurse in the first two hours after birth, they are less likely to be weaned early than babies who didn't nurse until four or more hours after they are born. This doesn't mean that the baby who needs special care (or is not able to nurse for some other reason) is doomed to breastfeeding failure, but it does point out that these babies and mothers may need some extra help in getting nursing established.

Often if the baby is held to the breast after birth it will nuzzle or lick at the nipple and not be interested in nursing. One researcher filmed a number of newborns who were simply placed, tummy down, on their mother's abdomens after they were born. The babies soon began to crawl on their stomachs towards the nearest breast. They found the nipple, then attached themselves and began sucking well without any assistance. The film involved only a small number of babies, but others have reported observing a similar self-attachment process with newborns.

Having the baby correctly positioned at the breast and latched on properly is extremely important for breastfeeding success. The best way for women to learn about breastfeeding positioning is to see lots of other mothers nursing their babies, but in our society few of us have that opportunity. (If you can attend La Leche League meetings during pregnancy, you

The baby doesn't have enough of the breast in his mouth. His gums are pressing mostly on the nipple instead of the milk ducts, which may result in less milk for him and sore nipples for his mom.

The baby has latched on well. He has taken a good part of the areola (the colored part of the nipple) into his wide-open mouth; his chin and nose are touching the breast and his lower lip is pressed down flat.

will learn a lot about breastfeeding just by seeing the other women with their babies.) The next best thing may be to have help from a knowledgeable caregiver or other breastfeeding expert.

Breastfeeding Techniques

When the baby shows interest in nursing—which can be right after birth or not for several hours—the mother should be helped to position the baby so that his stomach is against hers and his body is in a straight line, with his mouth level with her nipple. The most common position used for the first feeding is with the mother sitting upright with her back supported and a pillow on her lap to hold the baby up level with her breast. She supports the baby's head on her forearm, not quite in the crook of her elbow, tucks the baby's bottom arm around her waist and holds the breast nearest to the baby's head with her opposite hand. Her thumb should be on top of the breast and all the rest of her fingers below it, and well back from the areola (the dark area around the nipple).

The mother then gently strokes the baby's

lips with her nipple, and when he responds by moving towards the breast and opening his mouth wide, she moves him in close to the breast with her arm. She should "aim" her nipple towards the top of his mouth, to help get the baby's lower lip well below the nipple.

If this is done properly, it won't hurt. When the mother feels an initial painful tugging sensation on the nipple it means that the baby is trying to pull the nipple into position. She probably needs to either wait until the baby opens his mouth wider, or pull the baby in closer when he takes the nipple.

New mothers are often surprised to find that when the baby is correctly latched on both his nose and chin are touching the breast. They think the baby will suffocate (he won't) or that he is "too close" to the breast. (These mothers are probably thinking of all the bottle-fed babies they've seen who suck with just the bottle nipple between their lips and a large gap between the bottle and the baby's face.)

As the baby nurses, the mother should see and hear a changing pattern. It may begin with a series of rapid sucks, as the baby stimulates the milk to "let down" (move from the ducts further back in the breast, where it is made, to the ducts right behind the nipple so the baby can drink it). Then the mother should notice a suck, suck, pause, suck, pause or similar pattern, with the baby swallowing a mouthful of milk at each "pause." Eventually, the baby will change to a slower sucking pattern. If the baby continues with the fast "suck, suck, suck" pattern—no pauses or noticeable swallowing—he is probably not latched on correctly. The mother should slide her finger in the baby's mouth to break the suction and start over.

"This 'latching-on' thing isn't always easy," says Roberta. "When Germaine was born, he had such a tiny mouth and my nipple looked so big. I was so happy at the first couple of feedings when he started to suck, even though it hurt.

"But then the hospital lactation consultant came by to see how we were doing, and she said he wasn't on right. He was only getting a little of the milk, and my nipples were sore." Roberta learned to wait until Germaine opened his mouth really wide—"and that took some persistence because by this point he thought it was okay to nurse just on the end of my nipple"—and to make sure he was taking in part of the breast as well. "I knew when we got it right because it stopped hurting, and Germaine started to suck differently—I could tell he was getting a real mouthful of milk."

Feeding Times

The baby should nurse as long as she wants at each breast. When she is finished, she will either let go or fall asleep. Old recommendations that the baby should nurse for a certain number of minutes on each breast are not helpful. Studies have found that limiting the baby's time at the breast does not affect the number of mothers who develop sore or cracked nipples. However, when the length of feeding is restricted to a certain number of minutes, instead of until the baby stops on her own, many more mothers will wean their babies by the time they are six weeks old.

How often should the baby breastfeed? As often as she wants. Some babies may not nurse frequently during the first 24 hours, but nurse a lot once the mother's milk begins to come in. Some are eager nursers right from birth. As time goes on, many babies become more predictable, but some are always irregular in their feeding. The average time between feedings is about two or two and a half hours but there is considerable variation in this. Babies who are fed "on demand" gain weight more quickly and are not weaned as early as babies who are put on feeding schedules.

What about supplements of formula and water for the baby? Not only are these not necessary or helpful, they often lead to early weaning. Mothers whose babies are given routine supplements are five times as likely to quit breastfeeding within the first week as mothers whose babies are not supplemented. When mothers are given free samples of formula as part of a hospital gift pack, they are much more likely to give up breastfeeding before their babies are a month old. Using pacifiers, research shows, may also lead to early weaning.

Engorgement

"I felt like I had two large rocks on my chest," says Linda, remembering her experience with engorgement three days after her baby was born. "I couldn't bear to take a shower, it was so painful to have the water hit my breasts. And feedings were incredibly difficult."

The first milk the breasts produce, called colostrum, is made in small quantities and the mother's breasts remain soft for the first 48 hours or so after the baby is born. Then the "true milk" begins to arrive, and if milk production is over-enthusiastic ("I think my breasts thought I'd had twins," Linda says) and the milk is not removed, engorgement can be the result. The breasts become painfully swollen, both with milk and because of extra blood supply, and it is often difficult for the baby to latch on well.

The best prevention and treatment for engorgement is unrestricted breastfeeding—the baby nurses as often as he wants, for as long as he wants. This allows milk production to be adjusted to meet the baby's needs.

If engorgement does become a problem, some research has found that hand-expression of milk gives some relief to the mother. Other treatments, including ice packs or moist heat applications, may be helpful but have not been formally researched.

The Sleepy Baby

Some babies—especially those who have had a difficult birth, or who have jaundice—may be sleepier than usual. Bronwyn says, "My friends were envious because Talia slept so much, but it was a real problem. My breasts were so hard and full, and at every feeding I'd struggle to wake her up, somehow get her on the breast, and then she'd fall asleep again after about three sucks. I was so worried that she wouldn't get enough milk."

Bronwyn called a La Leche League leader who gave her some suggestions about getting the sleepy baby to nurse. "It helped to keep her close to me all the time, for two reasons. I could be alert to any signs of her starting to stir or wake up so that I could try feeding her. If I didn't pick her up when she started to make those little noises, often she'd go back to sleep again. Secondly, just me moving her from room to room and all our normal household noises kept her from going into such a deep sleep."

Bronwyn also learned some tips on keeping Talia awake during feedings. She undressed her—both to keep her a little bit cool and to provide more skin-to-skin contact—and changed her diaper before each feeding. If Talia dozed off at the breast, she would stroke under Talia's chin with her finger to encourage her to keep sucking. Rubbing the baby's feet also helped at times. Switching sides frequently—after every couple of minutes—was another method of keeping Talia awake and interested.

"It didn't take long before Talia was more wakeful and a better nurser," Bronwyn says, "and pretty soon there were days when I wished she was my sleepy baby again!"

The Fussy Baby

Jennifer's baby was the opposite of Talia. Michael slept very little and mostly took short catnaps, even during the first day after his birth, and he seemed to want to nurse 24 hours a day.

"And if he wasn't sleeping or nursing, he was crying," Jennifer says. "The first time I tried to feed him, he was screaming and it just seemed impossible to nurse him. I'd push my nipple into his mouth—it was open wide because he was crying so hard—and he didn't seem to notice it was there. He just kept screaming. After a couple of tries I started crying, too."

Jennifer's midwife showed her how to touch her little finger against the top of Michael's mouth. That would start him sucking, and help him to calm down. Once he was calm, Jennifer would quickly bring him to the breast again. If he didn't take the nipple readily, she would try touching either his lips with the nipple or touching the corner of his mouth. That would often encourage him to root for the nipple, and make it easier to feed him.

Do I Have Enough Milk?

Frightening stories in newspapers and on TV about breastfed babies who became seriously dehydrated have made new mothers even more anxious than usual about their milk supply. Most women who give up breastfeeding early say they didn't have enough milk. How common is this problem, and what can be done to make sure the baby is getting enough?

It's hard to tell what percentage of mothers are actually physically incapable of making enough milk for their babies, because many of the common routines (restricting the length and frequency of feedings, giving supplements and using pacifiers for babies) have the effect of reducing milk supply. Often when mothers who think they don't have enough milk learn to position their babies correctly and begin feeding "on demand" they find their milk production increases dramatically.

Other women become concerned about their milk supply because their babies nurse more frequently and sleep less than they had expected. "I didn't know that breastfeeding a new baby could be a full-time job!" says Lorraine. "Somewhere I had the idea that babies nurse for about 20 minutes every four hours or so, and you have the rest of the day to do what you want while they sleep. I had a whole list of projects I expected to take care of during the first month while my baby napped. When Matthew wanted to nurse every hour and a half, naturally I thought there must be something wrong with my milk. It helped to talk to some other mothers and find out that he was perfectly normal."

Some physicians have tried "test weighings" of babies to see if they are getting enough milk. This involves weighing the baby before and after a feeding and then calculating how much milk the baby has consumed. This is very inaccurate and not very helpful, because the amount of milk the baby takes at each feeding can vary quite dramatically. Research shows that when babies are routinely weighed before and after feedings, mothers are more likely to give up breastfeeding.

A better way to decide if the baby is getting enough milk is to observe the baby. Is he having at least one loose bowel movement each day (this may become less as the baby gets older) and at least six very wet diapers each day? Is he gaining weight? Is he active and lively and content? If you are concerned, contact your physician or midwife right away.

The Evidence About ..
BREASTFEEDING

Breastfeeding is the best food for babies. It provides protection against a number of illnesses. Breastfeeding is most easily established when the mother and baby are kept together from birth and the baby is nursed as often as she wants for as long as she wants. Supplementation with either formula or water and the use of pacifiers should be avoided.

Despite the strong evidence about the benefits of breastfeeding, our society makes it difficult for mothers to nurse their babies. Breastfeeding in public is often discouraged and mothers may have a hard time finding a private place for feedings. Our whole society would benefit from the lower medical costs and reduced strain on the environment if breastfeeding was truly supported.

Finding support and practical help with breastfeeding is often the key to success.

The World Health Organization recommends that breastfeeding be exclusive for the first six months, that solid foods may be added at that point but be only supplementary to breastmilk, and that breastfeeding should continue for two years or longer.

Conclusion

Making Decisions: Applying the Best Evidence

The experience of growing and giving birth to a baby is in some ways a simple process that, most of the time, works beautifully without any intervention at all. It is also a very complex process, with potential complications and challenging dilemmas. In Western societies, pregnancy and birth can be made more complex by the medical system, which has been designed to deal with those challenges—but which can, at times, get in the way of the simple and straightforward parts of pregnancy and birth.

A considerable amount of research has been done on pregnancy and birth, but it hasn't always produced clear answers. In some cases, the research has demonstrated that once-common routines are not helpful—as with electronic fetal monitors, episiotomies and shaving the mother's pubic hair. Some research has discovered lifesaving treatments—such as gammaglobulin for Rh negative mothers and corticosteroids for premature babies. Other research has only confirmed what women have always believed—that walking and moving around is helpful in labor, that having a support person

present is valuable and that women do know how and when to push their babies out.

The research, though, is only a foundation. It's up to you to decide how to apply the results of that research to your individual situation. This is your baby, your body, your family, and you are the ones who will live with the consequences of the decisions you make. You know what is important to you, and can make the best choices for your pregnancy, with the research results as only one factor (although certainly an important one) in the decision making.

Discussing Decisions with Your Caregiver

Florence was expecting her second baby. She'd had trouble breastfeeding her first, and was determined to get off to a better start this time. After seeing a video of newborns who were allowed to "self-attach" at the breast, she decided to ask her doctor to let her baby begin breastfeeding that way. She brought a copy of the research study to show the doctor.

"Well, there's a lot we have to do when the baby is first born, Florence," her doctor said. "The baby has to be suctioned, we have to check everything over, the baby has to have eye ointment. We can't just leave him or her lying on your stomach until he nurses—if that ever happens."

"In the video, they said the longest it ever took was one hour. Couldn't the eye ointment wait until after that?" Florence asked. "And couldn't you examine him while he's lying on me?"

"I guess so. I'll want to suction him first, and then I could put him on your abdomen. Really, though, I'm most concerned about the baby getting cold."

Florence thought back to the video she'd seen. "I think they used the heater that usually goes over the baby's incubator over both mother and baby. Could we do that?"

"I don't know if the equipment we have moves that way. I've never tried it." Her doctor sounded doubtful.

"Okay," said Florence. "I'll call labor and delivery and see what I can find out about getting a heater over me and the baby. I'll let you know what they say. And maybe after you've read this research, I'll lend you the video."

Florence was able to arrange for a heater to keep her and her newborn daughter warm. The baby lay on Florence's abdomen for about 10 minutes after birth, and then began to move towards her mother's breast. Before long, she had found the nipple and latched on beautifully. Florence was very pleased with the results of her decision.

Not all caregivers are as easy to talk to as Florence's doctor was. Some simply have a more intimidating way about them, and some are not interested in discussion.

Julie was less than pleased with the care her labor and delivery nurse provided. The nurse seemed impatient with Julie's slowly progress-ing labor and repeatedly told her to be quiet when she moaned during contractions. When Julie finally felt like pushing, the nurse seemed eager to get things over with.

Julie pushed as she felt the urge. She made a low moaning sound—almost a grunt—then took another breath.

"No, you're doing it wrong," the nurse said. "You have to hold your breath as long as you can and push as hard as you can, through the whole contraction. I want to see your face turn purple and your veins pop out." Julie was puzzled. This wasn't what she'd learned in prenatal classes or in the book she'd read.

"You've read that you shouldn't hold your breath too long, haven't you?" asked the nurse, noticing the expression on Julie's face. "Well, the books are wrong. I've been delivering babies for a long time, and the way to get them out is to hold your breath and push, push, push."

Julie thought back to what she'd read, and made a quick decision. She decided to ignore the nurse's instructions, and listen to what her body was telling her. When she felt the urge to push, and to hold her breath, she did. When she wanted to let the air out and take another breath, she did—even though the nurse was instructing her to keep holding her breath and push harder. It clearly was not a time to try to discuss it, so she simply kept her focus on the messages she was getting from her own body.

What can help you in discussing your options and your decisions with your doctor?

- Approach your doctor as a partner. He or she certainly has information and training that will be helpful in making decisions, and the two of you (or the three of you, since your partner may also be included) should work together to find the best choices for your situation.

- Ask lots of questions, but understand that your doctor won't always have the answers.

Many aspects of pregnancy and childbirth have not been researched; in other cases, the research has produced unclear or contradictory results.

- If your doctor recommends a certain course of action, ask why. Ask if he or she can direct you to any research studies or other sources of information. If your doctor seems offended or taken aback by your questions, explain that this is a significant decision for you and you want to know more about it.

- You can look up research yourself—either in books such as this one, in *Effective Care*, in medical journals or through the Internet—and bring it to the doctor to discuss.

- If your doctor is not supportive of your decisions, you can change doctors. This is not always easy to do, but may be your best option if you are really not compatible. You can also ask for a second opinion if a planned Caesarean or other major intervention is being recommended.

Liam's Birth: Decision Making in Action

How does this decision-making process work in real life? Each birth has its own challenges and each family has its own priorities.

Lenore has had five children, and a wide range of birth experiences—from a Caesarean section for a transverse lie to a planned home birth. You might think that by the fifth baby, there would be few surprises or issues left to deal with. Not so! Lenore's last labor and delivery—Liam's birth—involved perhaps more unexpected setbacks and decisions than any of his siblings. Here is Liam's birth story, which illustrates how women can play an active role in decision making—in partnership with their caregivers—even when labor doesn't go according to plan.

Lenore had planned a home birth. At her midwife's appointment just before her due date, she commented on how big the baby seemed to be getting, and the midwife suggested she do an internal examination since that can sometimes trigger labor. It worked. Lenore's water broke as she walked in the front door of her home.

"Labor started normally," Lenore said, "but as it continued, I kept feeling that the contractions weren't hard enough, weren't painful enough. It's hard to believe, but I wanted to feel more pain because I knew from experience that the contractions had to be more painful to get the baby born."

As the night went on, the midwives became concerned about Lenore's lack of progress. They encouraged her to walk, to sit on the toilet, to sit in the Jacuzzi, but she was still not dilating very quickly. They began to talk to Lenore about moving to the hospital.

"I didn't want to go, but I did understand their concerns," Lenore said. "Finally, at six in the morning, I agreed that we should go. It was just a gut feeling that something was not right."

When they arrived at the hospital, the midwives asked the obstetrician on call to examine Lenore. "The obstetrician said it was a big baby, I'd probably need a Caesarean and we might as well do it now. I said absolutely not. I'd had big babies before, and I wasn't ready to just give up on a vaginal birth. So she said I should have an IV with oxytocin to stimulate my labor and an epidural. If the baby wasn't out by noon, she wanted to do a Caesarean. I thanked her as politely as I could, and said we would like to talk things over alone."

Lenore discussed her options with her midwives and support people. "I decided I could take things one step at a time, that I didn't have to buy 'the whole package' right away." She decided she would have an IV and oxytocin, to see if stronger contractions would help.

But when the oxytocin was started, the baby's heart rate dropped drastically in response. "We had it turned off right away," Lenore said. Her contractions then stopped altogether—she thinks from the stress of the situation. Lenore knew she had to do something, so she asked to have the IV (with fluids, since she was a little dehydrated, but no oxytocin) put on a moveable pole and she headed into the shower—where she spent the next two or three hours.

"I felt safe in there. I could relax better. My contractions started again and then got quite strong. When I came out, my friend who was supporting me went around making the room as home-like as she could. She took down all the signs about epidurals, and she set out the blankets and sleepers we had brought for the baby. That really helped."

As the morning wore on, the midwife checked Lenore and found that she was fully dilated, but that the baby's head was very high. Lenore lay on her side and began to rock her pelvis back and forth, with her support people helping by pushing against her hip.

At noon, the obstetrician returned. She asked Lenore to move onto her back, and as she did, she felt the baby move down. "Then I pushed him out," Lenore says, "and it was a wonderful feeling. I lifted him up to my chest as he was born and didn't want to let go; I was just so glad he was born and everything was okay." The obstetrician was quite surprised, and said so. Liam weighed 10 lbs. 1 oz., and was home meeting his brothers and sisters an hour later.

Liam's story has an interesting sequel. Lenore explains: "We found out later that Liam had a serious heart defect, and he had to have major heart surgery when he was seven months old. I suspect that's why his heart rate dropped so dramatically when I was given oxytocin. I think, too, that this might have been just the right kind of labor for Liam—slow and easy—given his heart problem. I guess I'll always wonder about that.

"I used to be quite a shy, quiet person, but I've become much stronger, much more assertive, in part through my experiences giving birth," muses Lenore. "With each one, there were decisions and choices to be made. Some of the decisions I could make in advance, but you have to be prepared to deal with things as they come up." In a similar situation, you might make different choices than Lenore did—and those choices would be right for you.

Just the Beginning

When you decided to pick up this book and read it, you were taking responsibility for your own care, and for the health and well-being of your baby, during your pregnancy and birth.

However, this is just the beginning. As a parent, you will be responsible not only for decisions about your own life, but for your child as well. The decisions you make about how to care for and raise your child can affect that child for the rest of his life. All parents worry about making the right decisions for their children, and you will too.

You will have choices to make about how your baby is fed, who will take care of your baby if you work outside the home, what kind of diapers you will use, where your baby will sleep, how you will teach or discipline your child. You will have decisions to make about your child's medical care and education. It's a big—and sometimes overwhelming—responsibility. How will you know the right things to do? Just as with pregnancy and childbirth, you will work out the right choices for you, your baby and your family. These decisions may or may not be in step with the routines of your community. Any skills you can develop to help you be assertive in promoting your child's well-being will be tremendously helpful.

Your willingness to speak up and make decisions will benefit both other women having babies and the medical community. Women need to keep questioning whether medical procedures produce better outcomes, to keep asking why, to keep looking for better ways. Most of the changes—and many of them have been quite dramatic and substantial—in the way women are cared for during labor and birth have happened because women were determined to make their own decisions. The acceptance of vaginal births after Caesareans is one good example, and policies allowing fathers, doulas and other support people to be present at births is another. Most of these women had no thoughts of changing hospital policies—they just wanted to have the kind of birth experience that was important to them. But along the way they initiated changes that have benefited hundreds of other women—perhaps including you!

We hope that the memories of your pregnancy and your baby's birth will be positive ones, and that you will feel satisfaction in having made decisions that were right for you and your family. And as the arrival of your child leads you into the unique adventure of parenthood, we hope that your baby brings you as much joy and pleasure as our own children have given us.

Appendix I

Understanding Research Methods

Every pregnant woman is guaranteed to receive plenty of information and advice. Some of it is "old wives' tales"—stories that have been around for years. (One such tale, for example, advises pregnant women not to lift their arms over their heads, because that might make the umbilical cord wrap around the baby's neck. Mothers who've heard that warning are relieved to find out that this is physically impossible.) Other advice is based on the experience of the person sharing the information—or on something heard from "a friend of a friend." It might be interesting, but the individual experiences of others may not mean much for you and your pregnancy. Finally, there is information about pregnancy and birth that has been demonstrated or discovered through research.

Most of the studies discussed in this book have been summarized in *Effective Care in Pregnancy and Childbirth*, and the authors of that book carefully reviewed the research to see if it was valid.

What makes "good" research? How do you know when the results or conclusions from a particular study are likely to be meaningful?

The best, most reliable medical research includes:

- large numbers of people in the study, to reduce the risk that any benefits seen are simply chance or coincidence. This also allows for any rare or uncommon effects to be seen;
- a "control" group to be compared to the "treatment or intervention" group. The two groups need to be as similar as possible (except, of course, for the one aspect of medical care being treated). One way to achieve this is to assign the people coming into the study randomly to the two groups;
- a plan to eliminate bias as much as possible. The best way to do this is the "randomized, double-blind" study. In this kind of study, people are assigned randomly to either the control group or the intervention group, and neither the doctors caring for the people nor the researchers know who is in each group.

Two Non-randomized Studies

One study sought to compare home birth with hospital birth to determine which was safer. However, it included in the home birth group women who had their babies at home unattended, because they were too mentally ill or developmentally delayed to realize that they were pregnant or to get medical care. The hospital group all had prenatal care. Because these two groups were not comparable, the study was not meaningful.

Another non-randomized study compared two groups of women who had already had a Caesarean section. Some chose a repeat C-section for their next baby, while others chose to have a vaginal birth (VBAC). Because the two groups were otherwise very similar, researchers were able to show that VBAC is just as safe for the baby, and is safer for the mother, than a repeat Caesarean.

It isn't always possible to have all of these elements in a study, and that is especially true when it comes to pregnancy and childbirth. The "randomized, double-blind" type of study is most easily designed to research drugs. It's impossible to research something like the use of electronic fetal monitors during labor this way, because it will be quite obvious to everyone who is attached to a monitor and who isn't.

In evaluating research, it helps to be aware of some of the limitations of different approaches. For example, some studies compare the past to the present.

Before Caesarean sections could be done safely, almost all pregnant women with the placenta placed over the cervix (placenta previa) would die, along with their babies, when they went into labor. When these babies are delivered by Caesarean section, almost all the mothers and babies are fine. This is a clear example of a new treatment that worked and could easily be compared to past practice.

But comparisons between past and present are risky. Too many other things may have changed, as well as what is being studied, so that the "present" group is now very different from the "past" group of women.

Sometimes it is difficult to arrange for randomized studies. The people who are potential candidates may refuse to be randomly assigned to one group or the other, as they want to make their own choices. Some studies simply look at the results when people make these choices, and try to ensure that the groups being studied are as similar as possible.

Even when researchers try to set up randomized studies, there can be problems. People who are asked to be part of the study but choose not to be can affect the results—their absence may mean that an important group is being left out. People may also drop out part way through the study, and this can affect the results, making them less reliable.

Why is it important to know about these factors? You may read or hear about research results—but only when you know how the study was designed and carried out will you know if it is truly valid.

Meta-analysis: Combining Research Studies

When large studies have not been performed, sometimes the results of several smaller, well-designed studies are combined. Combining several studies in this way is called a meta-analysis. Meta-analyses are often used in medical research; however, with a meta-analysis one can never be sure that the results would be the same if a very large trial were actually done.

The results of research studies do not set up rules for the treatment of pregnant women. These studies give doctors a direction for giving women advice, and they give women a foundation for making decisions.

A meta-analysis combines all the possible errors in each small study as well as their results.

What Gets Researched?

Decisions about what to research are not based primarily on what pregnant women would like to know. There has been very little research on many areas of great concern and interest to pregnant women—nutrition during pregnancy, for example. Researchers are more likely to do studies on topics that are easy to study or that can readily find sponsors (drug companies, for example, sponsor a lot of research on drugs).

Evaluating Research

When the authors of *Effective Care in Pregnancy and Childbirth* were "studying the studies," they tried to eliminate all of those that were poorly done. Their book clearly notes the type of study on which the evidence is based, and how big the study was. We have relied heavily on their evidence and their evaluation of research studies in writing *Pregnancy and Birth*.

Two "Randomized" Studies: Not Reliable

Researchers wanted to find out if giving breastfed babies one bottle a day would lead to early weaning. They assigned breastfeeding mothers to either the "one-bottle-a-day" or the "no-bottles" group, and found that the babies in both groups weaned at about the same time. The problem with this study was that mothers who wanted to exclusively breastfeed refused to be part of the study, because they didn't want to risk being assigned to the "one-bottle-a-day" group. In fact, researchers found that the women in the "no-bottles" group were giving their babies as many bottles as the other group, and no conclusions could be made from the study.

In another study, researchers wanted to compare two approaches to handling babies who woke up and cried at night. Parents in one group were told to leave the baby to cry herself back to sleep; parents in the other group would go to the baby at night and offer comfort or feeding. After a few weeks, the researchers found that the "cry it out" babies were sleeping longer than the "comforted" babies. However, a high percentage of the parents in the "cry it out" group dropped out of the study—possibly those whose babies were sleeping less (and crying more). This makes it impossible to draw any meaningful conclusions from this study.

Appendix 2

Canadian Resource Organizations

PRENATAL / BIRTH RESOURCES

MIDWIFERY

To find a midwife in your area, start with your provincial association.

Prince Edward Island Midwives Association
P.O. Box 756, Cornwall, P.E.I. C0A 1H0
(902) 566-3102

New Brunswick Midwives
200 Inglewood Dr., Fredericton, N.B.
E3B 2K6

Association of Nova Scotia Midwives
P.O. Box 968, Wolfville, N.S. B0P 1X0
(902) 582-3151

Newfoundland & Labrador Midwives Association
132 Cumberland Cres., St. John's, Nfld.
A1B 3M5
(709) 739-6319

Association des Sage-femmes du Québec
54 blvd. Chambord, Lorraine, Que. J6Z 1P5
(514) 965-8673

Les Sage-femmes du Québec
BP 354, Station Côte-des-neiges,
Montréal, Que. H3S 2S6
(514) 738-8090

Association of Ontario Midwives
562 Eglinton Ave. E., Suite 102,
Toronto, Ont. M4P 1B9
(416) 481-2811
midwives@interlog.com

Association of Manitoba Midwives
Norwood Post Office, P.O. Box 83,
Winnipeg, Man. R2H 3B8
(204) 897-8672

Midwives Association of Saskatchewan
2836 Angus St., Regina, Sask. S4S 1N8
(306) 653-1349

Alberta Association of Midwives
1616, 20A St. N.W.,
Calgary, Alta. T2N 2L5
(403) 932-7777

Midwives Association of British Columbia
219-1675 West Eighth Ave.,
Vancouver, B.C. V6J 1V2
(604) 736-5976

North West Territories Community Health Centre
Keewatin Regional Health Board,
Rankin Inlet, N.W.T. X0C 0G0
(819) 645-2816

Yukon Midwives
39 Harbottle Rd.,
Whitehorse, Yukon Y1A 5T2

Doulas of North America
1100 23rd Ave. E.
Seattle, Washington, U.S.A. 98112
(206) 324-5440
Will provide a listing of Canadian members or
provincial representatives.

Motherisk Clinic
Hospital for Sick Children, Toronto
(416) 813-6780
Answers questions about risks to maternal and
fetal health during pregnancy. Caller leaves a message and a physician calls back. Also offers "warm
line" counseling for women experiencing nausea in
pregnancy:
(800) 436-8477

Centre for Addiction and Mental Health
33 Russel St., Toronto, Ont. M5S 2S1
(416) 595-6128
If you need help in giving up a drug, alcohol or
smoking habit, Assessment Services can help you
find services in your local community.

Infertility Awareness Association of Canada (IAAC)
Suite 206, 2378 Holly Lane
Ottawa, Ont. K1V 7P1
(800) 263-2929
IAAC provides information and support around
infertility. To receive their information package
($5) or to find your nearest support group, contact
IAAC at the above address.

POSTPARTUM SUPPORT

La Leche League Canada
18C Industrial Dr., Box 29
Chesterville, Ont. K0C 1H0
(613) 448-1842
There are La Leche League groups in most areas of
Canada, which provide trained mother-to-mother
breastfeeding support and monthly meetings. Also
offers a catalogue of books and leaflets, available
through La Leche League, on breastfeeding, parenting and child care.

Postpartum Adjustment Support Services (PASS-
CAN)
P.O. Box 7282, Station Main
Oakville, Ont. L6J 6L6
(905) 897-6262
Operated through Aid for New Mothers, PASS-
CAN links mothers with postpartum support
groups across Canada. An information kit on post-
partum depression is also available for $5. Runs
support groups and has a New Parent Information
Warmline:
(905) 535-2368.

Victorian Order of Nurses
(613) 233-5694
Private nursing service, sometimes covered by
provincial or private health plans with a doctor's
referral.

Canadian Association of Family Resource
Programs
101-30 Rosemount Ave.,
Ottawa, Ont. K1Y 1P4
(613) 728-3307/Fax: (613) 729-5421
Parent-child resource centers across the country
offer toy and book libraries, drop-in programs, parenting courses and support groups for new parents.
FRP Canada is the national association and can
direct you to the nearest center.

Mothers Are Women (MAW)
Box 4104, Station E
Ottawa, Ont. K1S 5B1
(613) 722-7851
Provides emotional support to women at home

through workshops, meetings and its quarterly magazine, *Homebase*. Subscriptions for *Homebase* are $25 and available through the above address.

One Parent Families Association of Canada (OPFA)
6979 Yonge St., Suite 203
Willowdale, Ont. M2M 3X9
(416) 226-0062
There are One Parent Families groups across Canada providing educational, recreational and social programs for single parents and their children. Each group produces its own newsletter outlining activities. OPFA can connect you with the nearest group.

Parents of Multiple Births Association of Canada (POMBA)
Box 234
Gormley, Ont.
L0H 1G0
(905) 888-0725
POMBA can put you in touch with parents of multiples births across Canada. It also publishes a newsletter and a variety of booklets on parenting multiples. Call or write for more information.

Infant and Toddler Safety Association (ITSA)
385 Fairway Rd. S., Suite 4A-230
Kitchener, Ont. N2C 2N9
(519) 570-0181
ITSA publishes a quarterly newsletter *Grow Safely* and Canadian subscriptions are $12/year. ITSA also offers several pamphlets and checklists on topics such as car seat safety and childproofing, which are designed to help parents keep their children safe.

GRIEF

Bereaved Families of Ontario
190 Brittania Rd. E., Unit 11
Mississauga, Ont. L47 1W6
(905) 507-2200
Runs groups across the province through local chapters.

The Compassionate Friends
685 William Ave.
Winnipeg, Man. R3E 0Z2
(204) 787-4896
Support organization for bereaved parents. Has over 60 chapters throughout the country, mostly outside Ontario.

Canadian Foundation for the Study of Infant Deaths
586 Eglinton Ave. E., Suite 308
Toronto, Ont. M4P 1P2
(800) END-SIDS or (416) 488-3260 (has a 24-hour answering service)
Provides information and support for grieving families through its self-help groups, which are offered across Canada.

BOOK SOURCES

Parentbooks
201 Harbord St.
Toronto, Ont. M5S 1H6
(416) 537-8334/Fax: (416) 537-9499
This specialized bookstore carries over 9,000 titles of books of interest to parents, teachers and other professionals on topics ranging from childbirth to teen pregnancy to family violence and self-help. Bibliographies are available and mail orders welcome.

Parry Sound Books
The Beatty Building
26 James Street
Parry Sound, Ont. P2A 1T5
(705) 746-7625/ Fax: (705) 746-4365
This bookstore has a broad collection of books for parents and educators on children with special needs of all kinds. Free catalog is available and mail orders accepted.

Great Expectations
A Canadian magazine for expectant parents. Ask at your caregiver's office or check your local library.

Index